Edward L. Hendrickson, MS

Designing, Implementing, and Managing Treatment Services for Individuals with Co-Occurring Mental Health and Substance Use Disorders
Blueprints for Action

Pre-publication
REVIEWS,
COMMENTARIES,
EVALUATIONS . . .

"**A**s more and more programs are engaged in improving services for individuals with co-occurring disorders, Hendrickson's second publication on this topic will have particular value. Unlike other publications, which focus on either overarching system planning or clinical services and practices, Mr. Hendrickson's work applies his twenty-five years of clinical program management experience in co-occurring disorders (COD) treatment programs to offer a wealth of down-to-earth, concrete, practical suggestions for real-world program directors, managers, and supervisors. He provides many examples, illustrating approaches to problem solving in program design, structure, and policy, and the most valuable sections of this book offer wonderful ideas for hiring, training, and supervising COD clinicians.

Although this book is focused on 'specialized' COD programs, it has potential value for program managers in any setting with COD clients."

Kenneth Minkoff, MD
Clinical Assistant Professor of Psychiatry, Harvard University;
Senior Systems Consultant, Zialogic

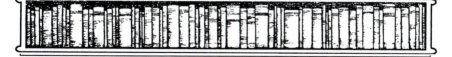

More pre-publication
REVIEWS, COMMENTARIES, EVALUATIONS . . .

"**H**endrickson has done a masterful job of providing in-depth advice about the practicalities of developing and running integrated treatment programs for persons with co-occurring disorders. This book provides useful guidance to policymakers, administrators, and clinical supervisors on establishing competent and effective co-occurring disorders treatment services; funding and efficiently using resources; staffing, designing, and managing treatment services, and evaluating and optimizing services. This book deserves a place on the shelf of all individuals involved in the development and management of services for treating persons with co-occurring disorders."

Kim T. Mueser, PhD
Professor,
Departments of Psychiatry
and Community and Family Medicine,
Dartmouth Medical School

The Haworth Press
New York • London • Oxford

NOTES FOR PROFESSIONAL LIBRARIANS AND LIBRARY USERS

This is an original book title published by The Haworth Press, Inc. Unless otherwise noted in specific chapters with attribution, materials in this book have not been previously published elsewhere in any format or language.

CONSERVATION AND PRESERVATION NOTES

All books published by The Haworth Press, Inc., and its imprints are printed on certified pH neutral, acid-free book grade paper. This paper meets the minimum requirements of American National Standard for Information Sciences-Permanence of Paper for Printed Material, ANSI Z39.48-1984.

Designing, Implementing, and Managing Treatment Services for Individuals with Co-Occurring Mental Health and Substance Use Disorders

Blueprints for Action

HAWORTH Addictions Treatment
F. Bruce Carruth, PhD
Senior Editor

New, Recent, and Forthcoming Titles:

Designing, Implementing, and Managing Treatment Services for Individuals with Co-Occurring Mental Health and Substance Use Disorders

Blueprints for Action

Edward L. Hendrickson, MS

The Haworth Press
New York • London • Oxford

For more information on this book or to order, visit
http://www.haworthpress.com/store/product.asp?sku=5471

or call 1-800-HAWORTH (800-429-6784) in the United States and Canada
or (607) 722-5857 outside the United States and Canada

or contact orders@HaworthPress.com

Published by

The Haworth Press, Inc., 10 Alice Street, Binghamton, NY 13904-1580.

PUBLISHER'S NOTE
The development, preparation, and publication of this work has been undertaken with great care. However, the Publisher, employees, editors, and agents of The Haworth Press are not responsible for any errors contained herein or for consequences that may ensue from use of materials or information contained in this work. The Haworth Press is committed to the dissemination of ideas and information according to the highest standards of intellectual freedom and the free exchange of ideas. Statements made and opinions expressed in this publication do not necessarily reflect the views of the Publisher, Directors, management, or staff of The Haworth Press, Inc., or an endorsement by them.

Cover design by Kerry E. Mack.

Library of Congress Cataloging-in-Publication Data

Hendrickson, Edward L.
   Designing, implementing, and managing treatment services for individuals with co-occurring mental health and substance use disorders : blueprints for action / Edward L. Hendrickson.
       p. cm.
   Includes bibliographical references and index.
   ISBN-13: 978-0-7890-1146-6 (hc. : alk. paper)
   ISBN-10: 0-7890-1146-8 (hc. : alk. paper)
   ISBN-13: 978-0-7890-1147-3 (pbk. : alk. paper)
   ISBN-10: 0-7890-1147-6 (pbk. : alk. paper)
   1. Dual diagnosis—Patients—Mental health services. 2. Dual diagnosis—Patients—Rehabilitation. 3. Mental health services—Administration. 4. Mental health planning. I. Title.
   [DNLM: 1. Mental Disorders—complications. 2. Substance-Related Disorders—complications. 3. Diagnosis, Dual (psychiatry) 4. Mental Disorders—therapy. 5. Mental Health Services—organization & administration. 6. Practice Management, Medical—organization & administration. 7. Substance-Related Disorders—therapy. WM 140 H498d 2005]
   RC564.68.H455 2005
   362.2'068—dc22
                                                                                        2005003810

CONTENTS

ABOUT THE AUTHOR

Edward L. Hendrickson, MS, LMFT, LSATP, practices in Alexandria, Virginia, providing treatment, supervision, training, and consultation in the area of substance abuse since 1971, and he has specialized in co-occurring disorders since 1982. For over two decades he has developed and supervised co-occurring disorders treatment services for Arlington County, Virginia. For over ten years Mr. Hendrickson served as co-chair of the Committee on Co-Occurring Disorders of the Metropolitan Washington Council of Governments, and he and a colleague received an achievement award from the National Association of Counties in 1991 for their work with clients with co-occurring disorders.

Preface

By the early 1990s most managers of mental health and substance abuse treatment systems acknowledged that they were encountering significant numbers of clients with co-occurring mental health and substance use disorders. This acknowledgment raised many difficult questions for the managers of these treatment systems. These questions concerned the following:

- *Mission:* Is it the program's mission to treat a co-occurring disorder?
- *Resource Utilization:* When limited treatment resources are available, which clients should be treated?
- *Staff Expertise:* Where will trained staff be found or what is the best way to train existing staff?
- *Design:* How should such co-occurring treatment services be organized and implemented?
- *Management:* How should programs be managed to ensure meeting licensure and reporting requirements, effective service flow, and other quality assurances?
- *Funding:* Where will the funds be found to pay for these services?
- *Effectiveness:* How will the programs and the community know if the services are effective and what are reasonable performance standards?

The purpose of this book is to create a single source for substance abuse and mental health professionals that provides a broad overview of each of these issues and suggests a variety of options concerning how each question might be answered.

The book is divided into three sections. The first section, composed of two chapters, examines the breadth, scope, and nature of co-occurring mental health and substance use disorders, provides an overview of the historical development of these services, and presents essential elements of effective treatment services for this population. Section II, composed of three chapters, examines the issues involved in developing treatment services for this population. The chapters of this section focus on identifying target populations, planning for co-occurring disorders treatment services, and examining the issues that might arise when these services are implemented. Section III includes five chapters and examines issues that commonly arise in the day-to-day management of such programs. The chapters of this section focus on hiring and training staff, providing clinical supervision, maintaining effective management strategies, operating in a larger system composed of other service and referral agencies, and ensuring the program's continued survival.

This book is intended to provide mental health and substance abuse professionals with an overview of common issues that arise during the design, implementation, and management of treatment services for individuals with co-occurring disorders and present strategies for dealing with them. In no way is this book intended to prescribe a single method of addressing these issues. Each community, treatment system, and client population is unique and must find its own solutions. However, this book is based on more than twenty years of experience that other colleagues and I have had in the development of such programs. It can provide readers with sample blueprints that they can use or modify when attempting to address these issues in their particular treatment system, agency, or program.

Section I:
From Then to Now—
From Where We Came to Where We Are

Much has changed in both how mental health and substance abuse disorders are viewed and treated during the past five decades. These changes have directly impacted the design of treatment programs and how such services are delivered. This section will review these changes, describe how these changes have impacted the development of treatment services and programs for individuals with co-occurring disorders, and present qualities that these programs must have if their services are to be effective. Chapter 1 reviews the development of the mental health and substance abuse treatment system in the United States and describes how treatment for co-occurring disorders has been slowly implemented into both systems. Chapter 2 provides an overview of eight essential qualities that a treatment program for individuals with co-occurring disorders must have. The purpose of this section is to provide the reader with the historical basis of our current dual treatment system and provide an overview of the essential philosophical tenets that an effective co-occurring disorder treatment program must follow.

Chapter 1

The Evolution of Treatment Services for Co-Occurring Disorders

HISTORY OF MENTAL HEALTH AND SUBSTANCE ABUSE TREATMENT SYSTEMS

In the past forty-five years a mental health and substance abuse information, treatment, and community support infrastructure has been created in the United States. Beginning in the mid-1960s, in addition to alcohol, nicotine, and caffeine, the use of many other drugs became commonplace. A much broader spectrum of society now used drugs such as marijuana, LSD, amphetamines, and barbiturates. New and much more effective medications to treat serious mental disorders were introduced. With the ability to better manage psychiatric symptoms through medication, many individuals were released from state hospitals and returned to the community, thus necessitating local community treatment outside of institutions. In addition, the entire cultural context of our society was changing; gender, racial, and other consciousness-raising and empowerment movements sparked an increase in the desire for self-growth and awareness. Therapies were introduced that focused on personal growth and involved the client equally in the change process. All of these forces exerted pressure on the limited existing mental health and substance abuse treatment resources and created the political will for the federal and state governments to begin to expand their systems of care.

Federal and state governments responded by enacting community mental health centers legislation that provided funds for community-based mental health and substance abuse treatment programs. The federal government also created the National Institute of Mental Health (NIMH), the National Institute of Drug Abuse (NIDA), and the National Institute of Alcohol Abuse and Alcoholism (NIAAA) to

provide funding, research, and national guidance concerning these issues. Most states soon followed and developed similar organizations.
New funding supported academic and paraprofessional training programs designed to equip staff with the knowledge and skills needed to
provide these new services. New professional titles such as "substance abuse counselor," "mental health worker," and "rehabilitation
counselor" evolved. In addition, the functions of professions such as
social work changed with the psychiatric social worker focusing
more on providing therapy than monitoring parent/child behaviors or
linking individuals with community services. Just as the federal government had separate institutes for mental health, alcohol abuse, and
drug abuse, so too did treatment programs become disability specific,
with separate funding streams at the state level. All of this activity
also spurred the creation of disability-specific treatment programs
that were supported by separate funding streams. Thus the new substance abuse and mental health systems evolved separately, each providing treatment for only one type of condition. At this point the concept of co-occurring disorders was still on the distant horizon.

During the 1970s, the movement of treatment from the state hospitals to the community meant that younger adults received most of
their treatment in outpatient settings rather than in hospitals. It also
meant that these young adults would no longer be isolated from their
peers, and thus, they would practice the same behaviors as others in
their age group. Hence individuals with major mental disorders began to use alcohol and drugs in unprecedented proportions. As the
youth of America grew alienated from mainstream society, many
never entered treatment but instead traveled around the nation or lived
in communes. Many were only partially treatment compliant and
many mixed alcohol and drugs with their medications. Mental health
and substance abuse programs seldom assessed clients for disorders
other than the ones that they were designed to treat, operating on the
belief that other conditions would terminate once the disorder being
treated was resolved. Neither treatment system was adequately
equipped to address the multiple needs of these individuals, and neither ventured far from narrowly defined views of etiology and
appropriate treatment strategies.

Furthermore, in most areas, the substance abuse treatment system
evolved separately as either alcohol or drug treatment programs. Alcohol treatment programs tended to encompass older clients who

used only alcohol, while drug treatment programs had younger clients who used a variety of drugs that usually included alcohol. Philosophically, individuals who viewed drug use as the result of some underlying psychological problem often ran outpatient drug treatment programs, whereas individuals who believed that alcoholism had a genetic and biological origin often ran alcohol treatment programs. Although many alcohol and drug abuse programs merged into a single treatment system for substance use disorders by the late 1970s and the biological etiology came to dominate the field's view, other systems did not merge until the 1990s.

THE BEGINNING OF CO-OCCURRING DISORDERS TREATMENT SERVICES

The publication of the American Psychiatric Association's *Diagnostic and Statistical Manual of Mental Disorders,* Third Edition (DSM-III) in 1980 created the framework for the development of services for individuals with co-occurring disorders. Unlike the previous editions of this manual, the DSM-III allowed multiple diagnoses for individuals. Hence an individual now could be diagnosed with a disorder such as major depression and, concurrently, could also be diagnosed with personality and substance use disorders. This meant that individuals receiving treatment in either the mental health or substance abuse treatment system could also have a disorder that would normally be treated by the other system.

In order to acknowledge the existence of co-occurring disorders, a term was needed to describe the phenomena. The term that initially came to dominate was *dual diagnosis.* This term was borrowed from the mental retardation field, which used it to describe individuals who had a mental retardation diagnosis and a co-occurring mental health disorder. However, that term was never satisfactory because it failed to fully describe the heterogeneity of the population who used alcohol and other drugs and had co-existing mental disorders. Other terms quickly evolved, such as dually disordered, mentally ill chemical abusers (MICA), substance abusing mentally ill (SAMI), mentally ill substance abusers (MISA), mentally ill chemical abusers and addicted (MICAA). These terms tended to describe only one segment of the population who had co-occurring disorders. Federal government agencies used the term *comorbid disorders,* but later changed the term to *co-occurring disorders,* which now has gained the widest acceptance. All of these terms continue to be used by treatment programs to describe their treatment population.

In 1987 a report by Ridgely, Osher, and Talbott, sponsored by NIMH, presented the results of site visits to programs across the country that had begun to provide treatment services for individuals with co-occurring disorders. The report reviewed the services of these programs and recommended that the co-occurring disorders be treated concurrently with either hybrid treatment programs using substance abuse and mental health staff or cooperative treatment arrangements made between substance abuse and mental health treatment programs. This report, plus a previous NIMH-sponsored one that reviewed the published literature on co-occurring disorders (Ridgely, Goldman, and Talbott, 1986) concluded that though treatment models in current use were promising, none was based on research outcomes.

As the dual diagnosis concept began to gain a foothold, treatment programs began to initiate services for individuals with co-occurring disorders. These initial services used either a sequential, parallel, or integrated model of treatment. The sequential services model advocated that one treatment program initiate treatment, and when that particular disorder was stabilized, the client would be referred to the other treatment program to complete treatment. For example, an individual with an alcohol dependence disorder and a co-occurring major depressive disorder would first be treated in a substance abuse treatment program. Once a stable abstinence was achieved, the individual would then be referred to a mental health program to address the depressive disorder. The parallel services model advocated using a mental health program to treat the mental health disorder and the substance abuse program to treat the substance use disorder concurrently, rather than sequentially. In the beginning, few programs initiated the integrated services model that designated certain staff to treat both disorders concurrently at a single treatment site because of a lack of trained staff and the incompatibility of such a philosophical model.

Sequential treatment was quickly found to be ineffective because it was very difficult to stabilize one disorder without stabilizing the other. Parallel treatment was not effective because it was difficult for an individual to concurrently participate in two different treatment programs in different locations that focused on different and sometimes conflicting treatment agendas. By the late 1980s, several integrated treatment models had been proposed (Hendrickson, 1988; Minkoff, 1989; Osher and Kofoed, 1989; Pepper and Ryglewicz, 1984), and by the mid-1990s it was generally accepted that integrated treatment was the most effective treatment model for this population. The report of a consensus conference convened by the federal government's Substance Abuse and Mental Health Services Administration (SAMHSA) on the treatment of co-occurring disorders (1998) concluded that integrated treatment was the treatment of choice for individuals with co-occurring disorders.

THE DEVELOPMENT OF INTEGRATED TREATMENT PROGRAMS

By the early 1990s, most community mental health and substance abuse treatment personnel accepted that individuals with co-occurring disorders were both in need of specialized services and were prevalent in significant numbers in their programs. Further, a growing number of professionals were specializing in treating this population. More and more conferences and articles focused on the treatment of individuals with co-occurring disorders. Also, by the mid-1990s, two major studies of the general population, the NIMH's Epidemiological Catchment Area (ECA) Study (Regier et al., 1990) and the National Co-Morbidity Study (Kessler et al., 1994), had documented that significant numbers of Americans had co-occurring disorders. A national awareness concerning the extent of co-occurring disorders and what was needed to treat them effectively had finally taken root.

However, although the integrated treatment model was now generally accepted as the most effective treatment approach for this substantial population, few programs had staff qualified to provide it. A study conducted by the Inspector General of Health and Human Services (1995) found that few staff felt they were adequately trained to effectively treat individuals with co-occurring disorders. Identifying the most effective treatment model also did not determine who should provide this integrated treatment and whether this integrated treatment should be offered in separate programs or be part of the existing substance abuse and mental health treatment systems.

Furthermore, funding also played an important part in the speed in which integrated treatment programs were developed. Even though the economy underwent unprecedented growth during most of the 1990s, the cost of health services was daunting to society. As a way of holding down costs, the amount and types of mental health and substance abuse treatment services that could be offered was often limited by managed care organizations or the lack of sufficient funding. The availability of services under a managed care system is totally based on what is authorized in the contract, and how well employees authorizing treatment services understand the specific treatment needs of an individual. Thus many contracts were developed that did not adequately provide for the full scope of treatment needed by individuals with co-occurring disorders, and few managed care companies had employees with expertise in the treatment needs of these individuals. In addition, because of the innate tug-of-war in a managed care system between cost savings and treatment need, the services authorized for an individual were not always based strictly on the treatment need. Thus, with a few exceptions, treatment services for the co-occurring disordered population had to be developed in the context of existing substance abuse and mental health treatment and funding resources.

Another trend in the 1990s that affected the quality of integrated services was the contracting out of many mental health and substance abuse treatment services to private providers. These public/private partnerships had mixed results. Many private programs were certainly less bureaucratic and less entrenched in the historical separateness of mental health and substance abuse services, thus making the development of integrated services easier. Mee-Lee (1994) suggests that, theoretically, managed care organizations have no historical reasons for keeping mental health and substance abuse services separate because they hate inefficiencies, and thus they can contribute to the availability of more integrated treatment. However, many of these program developers, in an effort to win the service contract, submitted bids that ensured low staff salaries. This meant that in most cases they had to hire less qualified or experienced treatment professionals. Thus, many programs that now had more bureaucratic flexibility still did not have treatment professionals with the expertise needed to effectively treat individuals with co-occurring disorders. Also, because governmental agencies had historically provided these services, systems that contracted these services out had few private entities from which to choose. Terminating a contract with a private agency would likely mean the elimination of services because no other qualified private programs were available.

Even though many barriers existed to the initiation of new programs for individuals with co-occurring disorders, many mental health and substance abuse treatment programs did add specialized services for these people to their treatment menu during the 1990s. This population was identified in significant numbers in both the criminal justice system and among the homeless. Regier and colleagues (1990) reported that a significant number of individuals in a prison setting had co-occurring substance use and mental health disorders. Pepper and Massaro (1992) reported that a transinstitutionalization had occurred for many individuals with mental disorders that resulted in their being placed in jails or prisons instead of state hospitals. They also believed that substance use among this group played a significant role in their incarceration. Several studies also documented significant numbers of individuals with co-occurring disorders in the homeless population (Drake, Osher, and Wallach, 1991; Herman, Galander, and Lifshutz, 1991; Fischer, 1991; Tessler and Dennis, 1989). By the mid-1990s many mental health and substance abuse treatment programs had begun developing working relationships with the criminal justice system and homeless service providers that included services for individuals with co-occurring disorders.

DEVELOPING THE NECESSARY INFRASTRUCTURE

In addition to the initiation of many new services in the 1990s for individuals with co-occurring disorders, other needs of the treatment infrastructure were developed. These included developing and identifying assessment instruments for this specific population; identifying the training needs of therapists working with this population and implementing such training activities; identifying subgroups of this population that had different treatment needs; developing treatment models designed specifically for this population; conducting research to document effective treatments; and publishing specific standards and best practices that provided treatment programs with guidance concerning which services to implement and evaluative tools to determine if they were following state-of-the-art practices.

The first assessment tool specifically designed for individuals with co-occurring disorders was introduced in 1992, and since that time several other instruments have been developed. In addition, research shed light on the effectiveness of other commonly used substance abuse assessment instruments for assessing substance use with individuals with co-occurring mental disorders. A review of assessment tools for this population can be found in Chapter 5 of Hendrickson, Schmal, and Ekleberry's (2004) *Treating Co-Occurring Disorders: A Handbook for Mental Health and Substance Abuse Professionals.*

In the 1990s, much effort also was expended in developing materials for increasing the knowledge and skills of mental health and substance abuse professionals who worked with clients with co-occurring disorders. Federal, state, and individual treatment agencies supported staff training programs; more and more national, regional, and local conferences focused on the topic; professional literature concerning effective treatment of this population made its way into professional journals and books; and videotapes were made for training purposes. As the number of professionals skilled in treating co-occurring disorders increased, they acted as supervisors and trainers for therapists without these skills.

Researchers and therapists quickly found that, in addition to being numerous, individuals with co-occurring disorders were far from a homogeneous group. It included individuals who had major substance use and mental health disorders that significantly impaired their ability to function independently, and individuals with less severe conditions who generally functioned fairly well in the community. The type and intensity of treatment offered to one client would not necessarily be appropriate for another client. As early as 1981 Pepper, Kirshner, and Ryglewicz reported that the substance use behaviors were different between younger and older individuals with major mental disorders. Since then a variety of subgroup models have been proposed with the quadrant model first proposed by Ries (1993) being the one most widely used today. A detailed description of these models can be found in Chapter 3.

With the acceptance of integrated treatment as the model of choice for this population, other intervention and client placement models were introduced that built on this foundation. Pepper (1995) proposed the community and client protection system model that advocated cooperative activities between the treatment and the criminal justice systems. Its purpose was to create a cooperative team composed of treatment experts and criminal justice professionals whose purpose was to ensure the safety of both the individual with co-occurring disorders and the community. The Phases of Treatment Model first proposed by Osher and Kofoed (1989) began to be widely used for client placement in the 1990s. This model identifies four treatment phases that clients pass through and proposes specific intervention strategies for each phase. This model was expanded into eight phases by Mueser and colleagues in 1995.

Outcome researchers also began to document effectiveness of treatment when modifications were made for the special needs of this population. In 1990, very few research articles had been published concerning the treatment of individuals with co-occurring disorders; however, by the end of the decade, well over fifty studies had been published in national journals, with many local communities completing their own studies on the effectiveness of their treatment services. A review of this outcome research can be found in Chapter 13 of Hendrickson, Schmal, and Ekleberry's (2004) *Treating Co-Occurring Disorders: A Handbook for Mental Health and Substance Abuse Professionals.*

Standardization of treatment approaches for individuals with co-occurring disorders began in the 1990s. The Center for Substance Abuse Treatment (CSAT) (1994a) published a *Treatment Improvement Protocol (TIP 9)* on providing treatment services for individuals with co-occurring disorders; this TIP became the most requested of the series, with an updated edition published in 2005 (TIP42). Furthermore, in 1998, the Center for Mental Health Services (CMHS) published standards of care for this population and the American Society of Addiction Medicine's (ASAM) criteria for substance abuse treatment placement ("Patient Placement Criteria, 2nd Revision" [2001]), now includes placement criteria for individuals with co-occurring disorders. Minkoff and Cline (2004) also have developed the Comprehensive Continuous Integrated System of Care (CCISC) Model, which helps mental health and substance abuse treatment systems develop the infrastructure to maintain a comprehensive and integrated system of care for all individuals with substance abuse and mental disorders. Initiatives to implement this model have been introduced at the state, regional, and local levels.

CURRENT CONDITIONS AND THE FUTURE

During the past twenty years the basic philosophical tenets, treatment models, and organizational structures have been identified that ensure effective treatment for individuals with co-occurring disorders. Many integrated treatment services have been developed and implemented and almost all mental health and substance abuse treatment professionals now accept the fact that numerous individuals with co-occurring disorders exist, and that they are in need of integrated treatment. The federal government, as well as many state governments have also begun to commit their resources to developing effective treatment systems. Substance Abuse and Mental Health Services Administration (SAMHSA), the federal agency responsible for funding and monitoring mental health and substance abuse treatment services, issued its Report to Congress in 2002. This report clearly documented the extensive prevalence of co-occurring mental health and substance use disorders in the United States and identified the important issues this presents for the nation's public health system and health policymakers. The report described a five-year blueprint for action that required SAMHSA to lead a national effort to ensure accountability, capacity, and effectiveness in the prevention, diagnosis, and treatment of co-occurring disorders. The report included numerous recommendations regarding funding, technical assistance, training, and research concerning effective treatment practices. Many states individually or in partnership with the federal government are currently initiating activities to increase the capacity of their mental health and substance abuse treatment systems to effectively treat this population.

However, in the early years of this millennium, many communities still lack basic services, and fewer still have a full range of services for those with co-occurring disorders throughout their entire continuum of care. Treatment is still often provided in a patchy and ineffective manner. Many mental health and substance abuse treatment professionals still lack necessary skills to treat this population effectively, and our universities are still not adequately preparing new professionals to treat individuals with co-occurring mental health and substance use disorders. Although great progress has been made in developing specialized services and training therapists to work with this population, much still needs to be accomplished. The purpose of this book is to provide a resource for individuals involved in the process of designing and developing programs for individuals with co-occurring disorders.

Chapter 2

Essential Qualities
of an Effective Treatment Program
for Co-Occurring Disorders

Treatment programs for individuals with co-occurring disorders come in all sizes and varieties. Their clients have differing levels of impairment. They operate in various components of the continuum of care. They exist as stand-alone treatment programs or as part of a larger treatment system, yet each must have certain basic qualities to be effective. These qualities include the following:

• easy accessibility to treatment services;
• treatment provided in an integrated manner;
• a competency-based view of clients;
• availability of a basic set of core services;
• flexibility of initial treatment requirements;
• variable lengths of stay;
• availability to a full continuum of care; and
• treatment services coordinated with other support services.

The purpose of this chapter is to examine each of these eight basic qualities.

ACCESSIBILITY OF SERVICES

Many individuals with co-occurring disorders participate in behaviors that are dangerous to both themselves and the community and most are ambivalent concerning treatment participation. Research has shown that treatment can significantly reduce these dangerous behaviors (Bartels and Drake, 1996; Bond et al., 1991; Drake, McHugo, and Noordsy, 1993; Drake et al., 1998; Durell et al., 1993; Hellerstein, Rosenthal, and Miner, 1995; Meisler et al., 1997; Mierlak et al., 1998). Hendrickson and Schmal (2000) also found that treatment retention was significantly associated with positive treatment outcomes for this population. This finding builds on similar findings for the general substance abusing treatment population (Hubbard et al., 1989; Hubbard et al., 1997; Simpson and Sells, 1982). Hence it is imperative that individuals with co-occurring disorders become engaged in treatment. Promoting treatment participation, however, is often a difficult task. Program design and philosophies contribute greatly toward creating a welcoming environment and easy access to services, both of which play a critical part in promoting client retention. A welcoming environment simply means fewer bureaucratic hoops that a client must jump through in order to receive services. Easy access to services means less time between a request for an assessment/intake appointment and the actual appointment. It also means that the location of the initial appointment will be at the same location as future services and that little delay occurs between the initial appointment and the first treatment session.

It has been my experience that the longer the delay between the initial request for service and the first service, the less likely a client will attend or be retained in treatment. I believe this is the result of two related factors. First, because the client is normally reluctant to enter treatment, the farther the initial meeting from the moment help is asked for, the greater the likelihood that denial and defense mechanism systems will be reestablished. When clients ask for help on their own it is normally the result of a moment of truth or a perceived crisis—both of which fade rapidly. Some clients are truly self-referred, but many will probably be referred by a third party, such as the legal system, social services, homeless services, the family, etc. Thus the second factor that affects referral is how responsive the treatment program is perceived to be by the person making the referral. Clients are much more likely to be referred for treatment when the services are believed to be easily accessible. Referring a client who is unmotivated for treatment requires the clinician to take a firm stand that the individual go for treatment, and then he or she must deal with the anger and resistance that this position normally generates from the client. When referring a resistant client the clinician wants to avoid the client coming back and complaining about having to provide significant amounts of information not easily available; take tests that the client sees no need for; or wait many weeks or even months before getting initial service. When that occurs, the referral agent often perceives that it is just not worth their effort to refer a client for treatment. Engagement in treatment is an important variable in predicting treatment success, and this engagement is strongly associated with minimal bureaucratic requirements and quickly receiving the first services.

INTEGRATED TREATMENT

Integrated treatment differs from sequential or parallel treatment. Sequential treatment involves treating one disorder at a time; parallel treatment involves treating both disorders concurrently but by different therapists or agencies. Integrated treatment means treating both the substance use and mental health disorders concurrently. The report of the National Consensus Conference, "Improving Treatment for Individuals with Co-Occurring Substance Abuse and Mental Health Disorders," held by SAMHSA (1998), recommended integrated treatment as most effective for individuals with co-occurring disorders. The CMHS (1998) report on standards of care for individuals with co-occurring disorders recommended that whenever possible, treatment of persons with complex comorbid disorders should be provided by individuals, teams, or programs with expertise in mental health and substance use disorders.

Four major principles are involved in providing effective integrated treatment. The first is observing and giving feedback to clients concerning how each disorder affects them and how each disorder can affect the symptoms of the other. For example, a therapist working with a client with alcohol dependence and dysthymic disorder points out how each disorder contributes to the client's financial and relationship problems. The therapist will also point out that although alcohol may initially reduce some of the client's depressive symptoms, these symptoms actually become worse the next day after drinking.

The second principle of integrated treatment uses the Gestalt concept of foreground and background; although the therapist is aware of how each disorder affects a client, he or she will not necessarily intervene with the same intensity with each disorder at a particular time. For example, a therapist has a client who reports serious suicidal thoughts and has a fairly detailed suicide plan. The therapist knows that this client has been using cocaine for several days and always gets much more depressed after cocaine use. At this point, the therapist will focus on the suicide risk (foreground) to ensure the client's safety. Once the acute risk of suicide is reduced the therapist will address the cocaine use (background).

The third principle of integrated treatment is to develop a service plan that has goals and objectives for both substance use and mental health disorders. If a therapist is treating a client with alcohol abuse and bipolar disorders, the service plan needs to include goals and measurable objectives for both disorders if the client's progress is to be accurately monitored. Minimally, these treatment goals include abstinence from alcohol and maintaining psychiatric stability. The objectives might include the client acknowledging the existence of both disorders and how they interact with each other; stating a desire to manage these disorders more effectively; achieving and maintaining abstinence, medication compliance, and so forth.

The final principle of integrated treatment is that all therapeutic interventions impact the symptoms of each of the client's disorders to some degree. Thus, the intervention should be designed to promote all the goals of a treatment plan and these goals should be monitored for both positive and negative effects. When working with a client with borderline personality and alcohol dependence disorders, a therapist may first have to help the client learn how to abstain from alcohol before accomplishing the treatment plan's objective of eliminating self-harm, because for this client drinking almost always precedes such an episode. On the other hand, another client who had only minimal alcohol involvement might significantly increase drinking once the episodes of self-harm are less frequent or eliminated. In summary, integrated treatment always involves seeing the entire picture but using wise choices concerning what to address and when to address it.

COMPETENCY-BASED VIEWPOINT

Most individuals with co-occurring disorders bring to treatment a life history filled with failures and often view themselves as incompetent to manage their lives effectively. It is not unusual for these individuals to be unable to identify a single strength. If they are to learn to manage their disorders effectively, these individuals must see themselves as having the necessary skills and abilities to do so. Thus programs providing treatment services for this population must promote competency-based client self-views. To accomplish this, treatment services need to have four qualities.

First, clients must be provided multiple opportunities to identify their existing strengths and skills. Intakes should include questions concerning what strengths clients perceive they have. When introducing themselves in a group, clients can be requested to identify strengths and skills they bring to the treatment process. When clients have made a positive change in behavior, they can be asked what strengths and skills they used to accomplish this feat. When a relapse occurs or an old behavior returns, the intervention can focus on what the client learned from the event that can be useful in preventing backsliding in the future. Essentially, the process of therapy focuses on what is right instead of what is wrong.

Second, a therapist never accepts "none" as an answer to the question of what strengths and skills the client brings to therapy. This is an important therapeutic stance because it communicates that the therapist views the client in a positive manner and believes that certain strengths and skills are present. Even though clients often perceive this position as inaccurate and naive, at some level it begins to instill a sense of optimism. A simple response to a client's position that he or she has no strengths or skills might be: "Well, you made it here today even though you feel very depressed and it takes a lot of effort." Without optimism, the necessary change cannot occur.

Third, the treatment program views any positive change as success. For example, a client with a long history of self-harm and alcohol dependence behaviors reports that for the first time she drank but did not cut herself. The competency-based response would focus on the fact that she did not cut, not on the fact that she drank. In fact, she would be praised for not cutting and asked what strengths and skills she had developed to accomplish this. Later it would be pointed out that she can use these same skills to interrupt her drinking, but at this point the total focus would be on the celebration of the changed behavior. This type of intervention is not meant to ignore real treatment needs but to positively reinforce changes that ultimately promote treatment success.

Fourth, treatment goals and intervention strategies are both realistic and achievable and designed to keep the client in treatment. Realistic treatment goals must be based on a client's initial capabilities. A client entering treatment with a long history of treatment failures, psychiatric symptoms not well controlled by medication, a history of substance use disorders since early adolescence and little leverage to keep him in treatment has very different capabilities than a client entering treatment with a court order, psychiatric symptoms that stabilize when medication compliant, and who has had significant periods of abstinence in the past. Using a competency-based focus, the goal of a treatment plan for the first client might simply be to see if he or she can be engaged in treatment, and intervention strategies might simply be case management and participation in a drop-in psychoeducation program. To expect more at this point in treatment would set up the client for another failure. However, for the second client, realistic and achievable goals could include regular participation in treatment, medication compliance and abstinence, and intervention strategies could include individual and group therapy, blood work and urinanaylsis to ensure abstinence and medication compliance, and participation in self-help recovery groups. Both intervention approaches are designed specifically for a client with a different level of self-perceived strength and skill competencies. By tailoring the treatment plan and intervention strategies to the client's perceived abilities, the likelihood of treatment retention is increased, thus promoting even greater skill development and awareness of strengths. Using a competency-based focus for clients with limited life successes greatly increases the chances of ultimately achieving treatment goals.

AVAILABILITY OF BASIC CORE SERVICES

All programs providing treatment services to individuals with co-occurring disorders will need to have available a specific set of core services if the basic therapeutic needs of clients are to be met. These core services include the following:

- psychiatric stabilization and detoxification services;
- medication services;
- psychoeducation programs that include a focus on the interaction of alcohol and other drugs and mental disorders;

- psychoeducation focusing on symptom management and relapse prevention needs of individuals with co-occurring disorders;
- individual, group, and family treatment modalities that concurrently address both substance use and the symptoms of other mental disorders;
- case management services that help clients effectively use other needed support services to address their various psychosocial and environmental problems;
- availability of drug-use testing devices, such as urine screens, breathalyzers, or hair samples; and
- knowledge of self-help groups and mental health recovery activities specifically designed for this population.

It is most effective when all these services are self-contained in the same program. However, realistically, psychiatric stabilization and detoxification services are normally provided in only one part of a treatment system's continuum of care.

Psychiatric stabilization and detoxification services are normally performed in inpatient settings, although detoxification is sometimes done on an outpatient basis and intensive residential settings are sometime used for psychiatric stabilization. Regardless of the setting, the goal of these services is to provide a safe and stable environment in which psychiatric and substance use symptoms are stabilized so that the individual can then participate effectively in ongoing treatment services.

Because most individuals with co-occurring disorders will need medication for their symptoms at some time during the treatment process, it is important that all programs providing services to this population have an on-site psychiatrist available for conducting psychiatric evaluations and prescribing medications. Depending on the size of the program, the psychiatrist may be a contract worker who is present a few hours a week, to a full-time employee of the program. In some cases this may also be a function of the program's manager who is also a psychiatrist. The psychiatrist must be knowledgeable concerning substance use and medications and be willing to work in a cooperative manner with nonmedical staff.

If individual, group, and family treatment is to be effective for this population, these services must be provided in an integrated manner.

The nature of integrated treatment was discussed earlier in this section and the manner in which case management services can be most effective for this population is described in the coordination of services portion of this section. Alcohol and drug use testing instruments need to be available to the staff for diagnostic and therapeutic reasons. The purpose for using these tests in treatment is not to catch someone in a lie, but instead to assess the extent of a client's use; validate the accuracy of client self-reports; provide material for therapeutic discussions; and occasionally, when based on a client request for extra support not to use. Alhough the results of these tests are often required in reports sent to referral agencies, the focus of these tests in treatment should always be viewed as therapeutic.

Finally, building a knowledge base of and referring clients to self-help recovery groups is an important task of treatment for this population. Though not available in all communities, many self-help groups have evolved over the recent years that focus on recovery from both substance use and mental disorders. Special interest groups can now be found in the Alcoholics Anonymous (AA) and Narcotics Anonymous (NA) communities and specialized groups such as Double Trouble and Dual Recovery Anonymous have built on the steps and traditions of these other self-help groups, offering meeting formats for individuals with co-occurring disorders. Staff providing these services must be knowledgeable about these groups, identify groups who would be friendly toward this population, and promote attendance by their clients. When these specialized groups are unavailable it is a tradition for programs treating this population to play an active role in their development by offering their facility as a meeting place or having staff identify clients who are capable of leading such a meeting and then providing them with the material and support necessary to establish these meetings. Depending on the functioning level of the clients served by the program, the support needed to start such a meeting might be limited to the following:

- suggesting where space might be found for the meeting and providing an Internet site for obtaining the material necessary to run a meeting;
- providing the space for the meeting in the program's facility during treatment hours;

- promoting client attendance; and
- providing a therapist who is available to provide support to the group leader before and after meetings.

FLEXIBILITY OF INITIAL
TREATMENT REQUIREMENTS

Each individual with co-occurring disorders entering treatment will have different treatment needs and different abilities and motivation to participate in treatment, thus a program providing services to this population must have the flexibility to vary treatment plans based on the specific needs and realities of a client. Treatment plans are always based on a compromise of the following: what the clients needs, what the client wants to do and is able to do, what the client can be talked into doing, and what services are available. As stated earlier in this chapter, long-term outcomes are significantly associated with treatment retention. Therefore, the initial treatment plan must take into consideration each of these issues and be designed to maximize the potential for client retention.

A client may enter treatment in need of alcohol and other drug detoxification, medication to ensure psychiatric stability, and residential treatment followed by long-term outpatient treatment and supportive housing services. Identifying treatment needs is the easiest part of treatment planning; the more difficult part is maximizing treatment services while promoting treatment retention. In this instance the client treatment needs are clearly defined; however, the client has no motivation to enter a detoxification facility and no third-party leverage to promote that level of treatment. The client does agree to have a psychiatric medication evaluation, accept some case management services, and attend an outpatient psychoeducation group that focuses on mental health and substance abuse topics. In such a case, programs providing co-occurring treatment services must have the flexibility to accept this limited treatment plan, at least initially. Placing additional treatment requirements on the client at that time may result in driving the client out of treatment.

In another case, a client may have the same treatment needs, but has a probation officer who will require the client to follow all treatment recommendations or be placed in jail. This client prefers treatment to incarceration, thus he or she accepts the more comprehensive treatment plan. Another variation of this scenario is that the client is willing to accept the full array of services, but no residential program is available to treat co-occurring disorders. In such an instance the treatment plan must provide the most comprehensive services available. In this case, detoxification would be followed by intensive (more than once a week) outpatient treatment. Although not the ideal, it does offer the client the most intensive treatment currently available. Because a full continuum of care is often not available for individuals with co-occurring disorders, the latter situation may be the norm.

VARIABLE LENGTHS OF STAY

To be effective, programs that provide services to this population must be able to adjust the length of treatment to the specific needs of the clients. Maximum treatment lengths often imposed by managed care organizations (MCOs) and substance abuse treatment programs have a tradition of requiring minimum lengths of stay because many of their clients enter treatment solely as a result of court requirements. Standardization is effective at controlling costs, helpful in planning for the number of annual treatment slots available, and reduces some of the resistance to treatment. However, it does not effectively deal with the complex and diverse needs of this population. If treatment services are to be effective, the issue of treatment length must be adequately addressed during the design or redesign phase of these treatment services.

Treatment services for this population or any other population do not have endless financial resources. The key to resolving the treatment length issue is to define a reasonable length of treatment for a specific subgroup of clients. The four subgroup models described in Chapter 1 can greatly assist service designers in their need to find a compromise between funding limitations, the need to plan for the number of clients that can be served, and providing services that will be effective. A realistic minimum treatment stay, combined with a program philosophy that allows the flexibility to either reduce or increase treatment length based on client progress can help ensure adequate treatment length while meeting the financial and planning realities that all programs face.

Again, the subgroup model in Chapter 1 can provide helpful guidance in this area. Because the model divides individuals with co-occurring disorders into four subgroups based on the level of their mental health and substance use symptoms, some assumptions can be made concerning length of treatment needs. Subgroup IV represents individuals with major mental illnesses and a substance dependence disorder (such as an individual with alcohol dependence and schizophrenia); Subgroup III represents individuals with a substance dependence disorder and a mental illness that results in lesser impairment (such as an individual with cocaine dependence and dysthymia disorders); Subgroup II represents individuals with a serious mental illness and a substance abuse disorder (such as an individual with bipolar and alcohol abuse disorders); and Subgroup I represents individuals with lesser psychiatric and substance abuse symptoms (such as individuals with generalized anxiety and cannabis abuse disorders). Generally speaking, the more intense the symptoms, the longer the needed treatment.

Clients in Subgroup IV will generally require the longest period of treatment, while clients in Subgroup I will normally require the shortest period of treatment. It is not unreasonable to use years in measuring the length of treatment that clients in Subgroup IV may need in certain parts of the continuum of care, such as outpatient or supportive housing. On the other hand, months may be an accurate measure of treatment length for clients in Subgroup I. Clients in Subgroups II and III will normally require longer treatment stays than if they had just a mental health or a substance use disorder; however their stays in co-occurring treatment services would be expected to be shorter than for clients in Subgroup IV. In addition, individuals in these two subgroups may also transfer to more traditional services and complete their treatment there once the less serious disorder is stabilized, thus reducing the length of time they participate in co-occurring treatment services. Using intensity of symptoms as a benchmark for estimating treatment length need and maintaining the flexibility to adjust treatment length based on individual progress are essential if high-quality service is to be achieved. It also provides programs with a reasonable measure that can be used to plan for both treatment slot and funding needs of a particular treatment population.

AVAILABILITY OF FULL CONTINUUM OF CARE

An important concept in both the mental health and substance abuse treatment fields is that clients may need different levels of care during their treatment and recovery careers. A client might begin a treatment career as an adolescent in an early intervention psycho-education program after being caught using a drug or participating in some other antisocial act. As a young adult, this individual may be in an outpatient treatment program for drug use and/or psychiatric symptoms. Later, symptom increases lead to placement in a substance abuse residential treatment program or a psychiatric hospital. Still later, this individual may be in need of a sober supportive housing or group home setting. These different levels of care are referred to as the *continuum of care*. Most clients will not need all of these services but some may need all services in order to achieve recovery.

Due to financial limitation, very few mental health and substance abuse treatment systems have a full continuum of care for their clients; and if they do, not enough treatment slots are available to meet all the needs at any given time. This situation is usually worse concerning the continuum of care for co-occurring disorders treatment services. However, even if the full continuum of services is not available, program staff must have a clear idea of what is needed if they are to develop a strategic plan for such a continuum of care. A comprehensive continuum of care for co-occurring disorders services includes the following:

- a prevention/early intervention component;
- an outpatient treatment component;
- detoxification/psychiatric stabilization component;
- a residential treatment component; and
- supportive housing component.

Prevention and early intervention activities have a long tradition in the substance abuse treatment field but are recent inclusions in the mental health field. A separate federal agency, the Center for Substance Abuse Prevention, provides funds for substance abuse prevention activities. Although no clear research shows that mental disorders can be prevented, early identification and intervention can result in reducing or eliminating the impact these disorders have on the individual and the community. Suicides can be prevented; negative effects on school and job performance can be greatly reduced; and the burdens that untreated disorders place on the community's social services, criminal justice, and family systems can be lessened. A clear relationship exists between nontreatment of certain of these disorders and increased risk of substance use disorders. The National Comorbidy Study (Kessler et al., 1994) found that 89 percent of individuals with mood and anxiety disorders reported the onset of their psychiatric symptoms on average four years prior to the onset of their substance use disorders. Since alcohol and other drugs reduce some of the symptoms of these disorders initially, it can be easily hypothesized that substance use disorders among this population can be reduced if psychiatric symptoms are effectively addressed. Several studies indicate a direct link between substance use disorders and attention-deficit/hyperactivity disorder (ADHD) (Biederman, 1999; Levin et al., 1998). These studies report that children treated for ADHD had significantly lower rates of substance use disorders than children not treated for their ADHD. Individuals with co-occurring disorders who are most appropriate for prevention and early intervention activities are those at risk of developing substance use or mental disorders. This portion of the continuum of care is usually the least costly and can help reduce treatment demands on the more expensive parts of the continuum.

Outpatient components of the continuum of care range from such activities as weekly group treatment sessions to daily intensive day treatment and include other interventions such as methadone maintenance, assertive community treatment teams, psychosocial support services, and supportive community living programs. The similarity among these services is that they are delivered to a client who is living in the community and participating in a wide variety of other life activities in addition to treatment. Individuals with co-occurring disorders who are most appropriate for these services are psychiatrically stable and can reasonably be expected to achieve abstinence in an outpatient setting. This component is the second least expensive portion of the continuum.

The other parts of the service continuum involve providing services to clients while they are housed within the treatment facility. These services include detoxification, psychiatric stabilization, residential treatment, and supportive housing. Detoxification is the process of managing the immediate physical and psychological symptoms resulting from the discontinuation of a drug. These programs may be hospital based or use a social detoxification format (i.e., a nonmedical residential facility). Many individuals can withdraw from most drugs without intensive medical monitoring (exceptions being withdrawal from certain sedatives and individuals with complicating medical conditions). These programs are appropriate for individuals who will experience major withdrawal symptoms once they discontinue their drug use or who need to demonstrate a drug-free state before entering treatment.

Psychiatric stabilization programs normally are found in hospitals and are used to help clients stabilize their psychiatric symptoms to the level that allows them to effectively live in the community. Non-hospital-based programs are also used by some communities to stabilize these symptoms and thus prevent hospitalization. Non-hospital-based programs are normally used for individuals whose symptoms are escalating but have not yet reached the level that would require hospitalization; hospitalization programs are designed for individuals who are so unstable that they cannot care for themselves in the community or who present a risk to themselves or others.

Residential treatment involves an intensive focus on all aspects of a client's life to help the client understand the causes and consequences of behaviors and begin to make changes in these behaviors. These programs are designed for individuals who are unable to achieve long-term abstinence and psychiatric stability in outpatient settings. The therapeutic community model which emphasizes self-responsibility is the most common model in use. Residents in these programs are encouraged to develop new ways of thinking and behaving toward their substance use and mental disorders. The model grew out of the Synanon Program, which began in California in the 1950s. Therapeutic communities usually involve treatment stays of three to six months or up to two years for persons with major substance use and mental disorders.

Supportive housing services provide a living environment that encourages both abstinence and psychiatric stability. These living environments normally have four to twelve residents and an on-site counselor who monitors the activities of the residents and provides ongoing support as needed. Mental health treatment systems normally refer to these services as *group homes* and substance abuse treatment systems normally call them *recovery* or *sober-living homes*. These programs are designed for individuals who need a stable housing arrangement to ensure their long-term stability and recovery. Supportive housing services for individuals with co-occurring disorders will need to ensure that any substance use is immediately addressed and that the use will not necessarily result in immediate removal from the program. The length of stay is usually based on how stable an individual is expected to become. For some individuals the stay may be as short as three to four months and for others it may involve years.

In reality, a full continuum of care will not be available for most individuals with co-occurring disorders, therefore the long-term strategic plan for programs providing services for this population will need to include goals and strategies for establishing a full continuum of services. Until that time, those services that are available must have enough flexibility to provide services for clients who may need a more intensive level of service.

COORDINATING WITH OTHER SUPPORT SERVICES

Many individuals with co-occurring disorders need additional support services to ensure their long-term recovery. These services include such items as financial aid, housing support, health concerns, employment supports, and spiritual resolution. In some cases these additional services are critically needed early in treatment, such as a stable and sober living environment, and some are needed later in treatment, such as job training. Regardless of when the services are utilized, there is a need to coordinate them with the direct treatment services so that the multiple treatment providers are extending consistent and compatible services to the client. Thus programs providing treatment to this population must include an active case management function in the service delivery plan.

Effective coordination goes beyond the simple act of referring clients to other services and determining if they are actually participating in that service. These linking and monitoring functions of case management are just a portion of effective service coordination. In addition, the therapist in charge of case management must also have sufficient knowledge of the services to be able to explain to the client why these services are needed for recovery at this time and what those services will involve; be able to establish a working relationship with the other professionals involved in the case that ensures all messages to a client are consistent and congruent with the treatment needs of that client; and possess the ability to advocate for inclusion or continuation of services when another agency is uncertain if the client is appropriate for them. This type of case management requires a program to allow staff sufficient time for performing these activities. Realistic caseloads must be assigned if case managers are to perform this function effectively.

CONCLUSION

Treatment programs for individuals with co-occurring disorders may be large or small, organized in various ways, and provide services for differing subgroups of this population. Eight basic qualities are needed if these services are to be effective. The next section of this book focuses on the issues involved in designing and implementing new treatment services for individuals with co-occurring disorders.

Section II:
Getting Started—
Creating New Programs
or Expanding Existing Ones

Creating a new program or expanding service capability within an existing one in order to initiate treatment services for individuals with co-occurring disorders requires a great deal of forethought and planning. Individuals with co-occurring disorders are a very heterogeneous population and thus have a wide variety of treatment and other support service needs. These treatment variations must be taken into consideration when planning for and implementing services. This section of the book reviews the essential issues that need to be addressed and the decisions that need to be made when designing and implementing these new treatment services. Chapter 3 provides methods for addressing the heterogeneity of this treatment population that can assist planners in defining the target individuals for these new services. Chapter 4 describes the issues involved in the design of these new services, and Chapter 5 examines the numerous issues that program developers face when implementing these new services in different types of programs. The purpose of this section is to provide readers with guideposts in their efforts to design and implement new treatment services for this population; to warn of potential problems if certain design and implementation issues are not planned for adequately; but foremost, to demonstrate that treatment services can be implemented effectively when certain steps are taken in a thoughtful manner.

Chapter 3

Identifying a Target Population

Numerous studies of substance abuse and mental health treatment populations and two major studies of the general population document significant rates of co-occurrence of substance use with certain other mental disorders. Studies of substance abuse treatment populations indicate 60 percent or greater co-occurrence rates when personality disorders are included (Nace, 1989; Powell et al., 1982; Ross, Glaser, and Germanson, 1988; Weissman, Myers, and Harding, 1980); studies of mental health treatment populations indicate co-occurrence rates of 40 to 50 percent (Ananth, 1989; Caton et al., 1989; Drake and Wallach, 1989; Ridgely, Goldman, and Talbott, 1986). Regier and colleagues (1990) presented the first major study of co-occurrence of substance use and mental disorders in the general population. They examined the National Institute of Mental Health's Epidemiologic Catchment Area (ECA) Study and found that 29 percent of individuals with a mental disorder also had a substance use disorder; 37 percent of individuals with an alcohol disorder also had a mental disorder; and 53 percent of individuals with a drug disorder other than alcohol also had a mental disorder. They also found that individuals with co-occurring disorders were twice as likely to be in treatment for at least one of their disorders. The National Longitudinal Alcohol Epidemiologic Study (NLAES), sponsored by the National Institute of Alcohol Abuse and Alcoholism (NIAAA) also found that individuals with alcohol use disorders and co-occurring mental disorders were much more likely to be in treatment than individuals with just alcohol disorders (Onken et al., 1997). The results of the National Comorbidity Study reported by Kessler and colleagues (1994) found that 51 percent of individuals with a mental disorder also experienced a substance use disorder during their lifetime, and 41 to 66 percent of individuals with a substance use disorder experienced a mental disorder sometime in their lives. Those with alcohol abuse disorder had the lowest level of co-occurrence, and individuals with drug dependency disorders experienced the greatest level of co-occurrence. This study also indicated that individuals with dependency and co-occurring mental disorders were much more likely to be in treatment than individuals with just one disorder.

These results, other research findings, and the realities of providing substance abuse and mental health treatment services have created a national consensus that specialized treatment services are needed for this population. However, few if any of our mental health and substance abuse treatment systems currently have these specialized services available in their full continuums of care. This situation has created substantial internal and external pressure to develop these specialized services. One of the problems facing those involved in developing the new services is that this treatment population is very diverse and does not represent a single group with similar needs. Clients in need of these services have different levels of involvement with alcohol and other drugs; different levels of psychiatric symptoms; different levels of functional impairment, and thus different treatment needs. When planning services, therefore, the first decision must determine for which group of individuals these services will be designed. This chapter will address the following issues:

- discuss this heterogeneity in detail;
- present subgroup models that have been proposed for this population;
- recommend the most effective subgroup model in planning services for this population;
- present a needs assessment tool that communities can use to identify gaps in services that incorporates this subgroup model;
- discuss how the information obtained from the needs assessment can be used to determine the target population for these new services; and
- describe a method for ensuring that all needed services are clearly identified and an implementation plan created.

HETEROGENEITY OF CO-OCCURRING DISORDERS TREATMENT POPULATIONS

The heterogeneity of this population results from how the interaction of substance use and psychiatric symptoms impacts an individual's ability to care for self and live independently in the community. Normally, the more extensive the use of alcohol and drugs, the greater the impact this use has on the individual; likewise, the more serious the mental disorder, the more it impacts the individual. However, that is not always the case. For example, an individual with bipolar disorder may be symptom free for extended periods; when symptomatic, the medication works to minimize symptoms. Another individual with the same disorder may have constant symptoms that are not well maintained by medication. Also, two individuals, both with alcohol dependence disorders and who drink heavily on a daily basis, may function at very different levels. One may hold a job, perform many of his family responsibilities, and in general be a productive citizen, whereas the other individual may be homeless, unable to maintain significant relationships, and require extensive supports from the community.

Although each disorder has its unique impact, multiple disorders also interact to create an equally unique effect on each individual. For example, an individual might have a dysthymic disorder well controlled by medication, but when he or she uses cocaine the symptoms become those of a major depressive disorder which the medication does not control and hence the desire to use cocaine increases. Either disorder alone will not have the same impact on this individual's level of functioning as will both disorders interacting. Thus the interactions between disorders contribute even further to the heterogeneity of the population.

Although each individual experiences a unique impact from his or her substance use and mental disorders, it is possible to categorize by intensity of symptoms. Doing so allows for the development of subgroup models. Such models are necessary for planners, managers, and clinicians who must answer the questions *Which clients can be treated together?* and *What level of services do they need?* The next section reviews the proposed subgroup models for this population. Recommendations are made concerning which model appears to be most useful currently.

USEFUL SUBGROUP MODELS FOR THIS POPULATION

Individuals with co-occurring disorders represent a varied population that complicates the treatment planning process. Pepper, Kirshner, and Ryglewicz (1981) divided individuals with serious mental disorders into two subgroups: younger individuals who used alcohol and drugs and had spent little time in state hospitals and an older group that used only alcohol, if they used at all, and had spent significant time in psychiatric hospitals. Schuckit (1985) based his subgroups on the onset of psychiatric symptoms in an attempt to differentiate substance-induced disorders from co-occurring disorders. Cloninger (1987) described Type I alcoholics who had a later onset of the alcohol dependence disorder with little other pathology in the family, and defined Type II as those who had an early onset of alcohol dependence with one or both parents demonstrating antisocial behaviors.

As the understanding of this population grew, other subgroup models were introduced, reflecting an increase in knowledge about the variety of considerations needed for effective treatment planning. Blackwell, Beresford, and Lambert (1988) proposed a five-subgroup model that was based on the presence of alcohol and/or psychiatric disorders. Sandberg, Greenberg, and Birkmann (1991) proposed four subgroups of individuals with co-occurring disorders based on why they used alcohol and drugs. Lehman (1996) proposed a five-subgroup model based on the types of substance use disorders, mental health disorders, medical problems, and social problems that affected the client. Hien and colleagues (1997) proposed a three-subgroup model based on which disorder was primary.

The subgroup models found most helpful in managing multifarious caseloads are based on the intensity of an individual's substance use and psychiatric symptoms. Two such models have been proposed, one by Ries (1993) and the other by the Metropolitan Washington Council of Governments (1995) (see Table 3.1). The advantage of these models is that they are based on the level of symptoms and the impact of these symptoms on the individual. As discussed previously, the same disorder can affect individuals in many different ways, thus basing treatment subgroups primarily on the types of disorders present often does not increase the homogeneity of this population. Again, an individual with an alcohol dependency disorder and

TABLE 3.1. Subgroup Models

Ries Subgroup Model	COG Subgroup Model	MH Symptoms	SA Symptoms
1	3	Low	Low
3	2	Low	High
2	4	High	Low
4	1	High	High

a major depressive disorder might have only short periods when depressive and alcohol symptoms are present. This individual might have a job, a family, and might be fairly self-sufficient. Another individual with the same disorders might be symptomatic for extensive periods and thus be unable to hold a job, maintain intimate relationships, or have a peer support network. The level of symptoms and the ability to function independently are very different for these individuals.

Again, the two important questions that need to be answered when planning services for this population are *Which clients can be treated together?* and *What level of services do they need?* My experience shows that functioning level provides the best information for answering these questions. In general, the functioning level is best predicted by the intensity of the client's symptoms as discussed in the previous two models. No current subgroup model can ensure the accurate identification of all treatment needs for each client in that subgroup. I believe the four-subgroup model proposed by Ries, which is the subgroup model most used currently, can be effectively used in the development of need-assessment tools for this population and can help determine which clients would be most effectively served by a particular program.

DESIGNING AND CONDUCTING A NEEDS ASSESSMENT

Needs assessments for co-occurring disorders treatment services must determine which types of substance use, mental health, and co-occurring disorders treatment services are currently being offered; in which parts of the system's continuum of care these services are being offered; and which types of clients they are being offered to. In addition, the needs assessment must identify the number of clients who are in need of co-occurring disorders treatment services. Once treatment service data is collected and compiled, it can be compared with actual needs. The gap between services currently offered and services needed helps focus the discussion on which new services need to be added. The purpose of this section is to discuss how to conduct an effective needs assessment of treatment services for individuals with co-occurring disorders and present a needs-assessment tool that can be used or modified by communities conducting such assessments of their treatment systems.

The first step in developing a needs-assessment tool for measuring existing treatment services for individuals with co-occurring disorders is to ensure that the heterogeneity of this population is reflected accurately in the instrument. I believe that Ries's four subgroups mentioned in the previous section are currently the best model for this purpose. Because symptom level is predictive of treatment needs and functioning level for most individuals, using this model helps compare current treatment services with those who can actually use these services. For example, there may be residential treatment that provides integrated substance use and mental health treatment for clients who are psychiatrically stable and can handle some level of confrontation, but no such services are available for individuals who cannot be fully stabilized psychiatrically. A needs assessment that just examines available services and where the services are offered will not determine if all segments of the co-occurring disorders population can use these services.

The main part of the needs assessment will focus on types of services being currently offered and location of those services. Chapter 2 identified basic core treatment services that range from detoxification and psychiatric stabilization to different forms of outpatient treatment that all individuals with co-occurring disorders may be in need of, thus each of these services needs to be included in the survey instrument. Likewise, Chapter 2 also identified the various components of the continuum of care that this population may need to utilize during their treatment careers that range from prevention/early intervention activities to supportive housing. Any needs assessment for this population should also collect data concerning the availability of these components. Finally, the needs assessment must also determine if the current services have the other qualities of effective co-occurring disorders treatment services mentioned in Chapter 2 and if the treatment capacity of these services adequately meets the number of clients who need them. Appendix A contains a model needs-assessment instrument for this population that promotes the collection of all the information previously mentioned that can be used as is or modified by communities conducting such surveys.

In order to compare what treatment services are actually available to the level of need for these services requires that a community have some reasonable estimate of the number of its citizens in need of such services. Several methods can be used to determine this estimate. The first is to include a question on the needs assessment concerning each program's estimate of the number of current clients who have co-occurring disorders. The question can further inquire the number that would need dual-diagnosis capable or dual-diagnosis enhanced treatment as defined by the American Society of Addiction Medicine (ASAM PC-2R, 2001). Dual-diagnosis capable services are defined as additions to a traditional substance abuse or mental health program that allow the staff to treat less-impaired individuals with co-occurring disorders, such as medication services being added to a substance abuse program or a substance abuse psychoeducation group being added to a mental health program. Dual-diagnosis enhanced services are targeted for individuals with severe mental health and substance abuse symptoms and thus such programs are capable of treating unstable and severely impaired individuals. Using this model helps discern into which subgroups these clients might fall. These reported percentages can then be compared to studies of similar mental health and substance abuse treatment programs to gain some sense of the accuracy of the reported numbers. Table 3.2 summarizes research findings concerning the number of clients with co-occurring disorders that have been found in various types of mental health and substance abuse treatment programs. In addition, not all individuals with co-occurring disorders in a community are found in treatment programs, as shown by the results of two large national studies that examined the prevalence of co-occurring disorders in the general population, presented in Table 3.2. This information can be used with a community's census figures to estimate the number of individuals in that community who might need co-occurring disorders treatment services at any given time. Using either method, or better, using a

TABLE 3.2. Percentage of Individuals with Co-Occurring Disorders

Studies	Findings
General Population	3-4% of individuals living in the community at any time will have co-occurring disorders
Mental Health Tx Programs	40-60% of individuals in treatment had a co-occurring substance use disorder
Substance Abuse Tx Programs	50-60% of individuals in treatment had a co-occurring mental health disorder

combination of both, can provide reasonable estimates of the number of individuals who are in need of co-occurring disorders treatment services.

The process by which the survey will be conducted is as important as the needs-assessment tool and estimates of individuals in need. Before a successful needs assessment can be conducted it must be sponsored by some organization in the community that has the respect of all those who will be surveyed. Without this element of respect, those conducting the assessment may not obtain access to the individuals who need to be interviewed or they may be unable to get the necessary information. The community organization must be viewed as having the best interests of the clients and the community at heart; be knowledgeable about this population and capable of conducting such a survey; and be able to report fair and impartial findings. Normally the best approach for such a needs assessment is that sponsorship be conducted by some coordinating body such as the community mental health association or a local planning council. Once the sponsorship has been identified, a coordinating body that includes all the agencies and important individuals in the community who could be impacted by the needs-assessment findings should be invited to participate in planning the survey. At a minimum, the coordinating body should include individuals from the mental health and substance abuse treatment community; health care system; social services system; criminal justice system; and community advocates for the treatment of substance use and mental disorders. Keep in mind when selecting these individuals that they later may become important advocates for the survey's findings.

Once the sponsoring agency and the survey's coordinating body have been identified, the next step is to determine which programs will be surveyed. Essentially all programs that provide mental health, substance abuse, or co-occurring disorders treatment services need to be included in the needs-assessment process. This includes public and private programs and programs outside the community that clients use, such as a regional hospital, residential treatment center, or detoxification program. Also it must be decided who is the most appropriate person to speak with at each of these facilities to obtain needed information and what is the most appropriate way to request participation in the survey. Members of the coordinating body of this survey will be invaluable resources in helping to answer these questions.

The final step in this assessment process involves determining who will actually conduct the survey. Depending on the size of the systems being surveyed and the funding availability, the assessment might be conducted by a private consulting firm or by professionals currently working in the systems being surveyed. Regardless of who is selected to do the needs assessment, they too must be perceived as being unbiased toward any programs and to be knowledgeable concerning treatment of this population if doors are to open and information is to be made readily available. Thus, consulting firms conducting such surveys will need to have a mental health and/or substance abuse track record and must have consultants who are knowledgeable about these services. If professionals from existing agencies are used, I would recommend that a two-person team minimum be used to conduct the survey. Such a team should include at least one mental health and one substance abuse professional. These professionals must also have a clear understanding of how the system that they do not represent operates, what issues it faces, and by what values it operates. To add both creditability and a broad focus to the team I would also recommend that these individuals currently be part of a management team in their specific programs, but also have strong clinical backgrounds. Ultimately, the ability to conduct an effective needs assessment will depend a great deal on the personalities and the understandings that those individuals conducting the survey bring to the process. Once the survey is completed, the data must then be analyzed and decisions made concerning which services will be developed and when.

ANALYZING THE FINDINGS, MAKING DECISIONS, AND DEVELOPING A STRATEGY

Once the needs assessment has been completed, the collected data must be analyzed. A decision must be made concerning who the target population will be and what type of services will be offered, and a strategy must be developed for meeting needs identified by the survey that will not be addressed by these new services. The data analysis part of this process must answer the four following important questions:

1. Which co-occurring treatment services are currently being provided to which subgroups?
2. In what parts of the continuum of care are these co-occurring treatment services being provided?
3. Do these services have the essential qualities of effective co-occurring disorders treatment services?
4. Are they sufficient in number to meet the community's treatment needs?

Once these questions are answered, the community will be able to identify the gaps that exist between what is currently being offered and what is ultimately needed. Appendix A includes a format titled Existing Community Co-Occurring Disorders Treatment Resources that is designed to organize the data collected by the Model Needs Assessment in such a manner that service gaps are easily identified.

Once the analysis of the needs assessment is completed, the task of the survey's coordinating body is to decide which new services will be implemented and for whom. This decision will ultimately be based on a variety of the following factors:

- what is needed;
- what services would be most easily implemented;
- cost of these new services;
- cost to the community for not implementing these new services;
- flexibility and willingness of existing programs to implement or support these new services;
- staff skill levels and training availability; and
- level of political and professional support for different types of services.

Many factors must be taken into consideration by this decision-making process, however, the ultimate goal should be how to provide the greatest number of clients in need with the greatest number of new treatment services. The following examples describe how this decision-making process might unfold.

In one community, the needs assessment identified that individuals in Subgroups I, III, and IV were found in the substance abuse treatment programs and individuals in Subgroups, I, II, and IV were found in mental health treatment programs; however, none of these programs provided specialized co-occurring disorders treatment services for them. In addition, neither the substance abuse nor the mental health treatment systems had a complete continuum of care. The substance abuse treatment system lacked a residential treatment component and the mental health system lacked a supportive housing component. The decision-making process in this case centered on how to initiate these co-occurring disorders treatment services. In essence, this community began from scratch, so there was a need to implement these new services in all components of the existing continuums of care. Initially there was some resistance to spending new money on these services before a full continuum of care of mental health and substance abuse services was completed. However, it was finally acknowledged that since these clients are already in the treatment programs, their special needs should be addressed. Since little money was available to expand these services, it was decided to provide the new services to the subgroup who currently had the most negative impact on the community. It was decided that Subgroup IV would be the target population because the mixture of substance use with serious mental disorders caused substantial demands on the community criminal justice, health care, and social service systems. The mental health system finally agreed to provide outpatient co-occurring disorders treatment services with funds designated for this purpose. Furthermore, the substance abuse treatment system agreed to allow these individuals to participate in its short-term detoxification program as long as they did not need psychiatric hospitalization. The local mental health advocacy groups also supported the initiation of these services in the mental health system. The final step in the process was to develop a plan for implementing co-occurring disorders treatment services in all other parts of the existing continuums of care and incorporating these services in any existing plan to add residential or supportive housing to the continuums of care.

In another community, the needs assessment found that both the mental health and substance abuse treatment systems had a complete continuum of care for their clients. The substance abuse treatment system provided specialized co-occurring disorders treatment services in all parts of its continuum of care to individuals in Subgroups I and III, but did not accept anyone with a serious mental disorder. In addition, the mental health treatment system provided no co-occurring disorders treatment services for the clients who used alcohol and other drugs. The decision-making process in this case centered on how to implement co-occurring treatment services for individuals with serious mental disorders. In this community, both the mental health and substance abuse systems remained resistant to implementing such services; thus it was decided to initiate a new program to provide these services. Because new funds were limited and the start-up cost of a new program was greater than the cost of expanding existing services, it was further decided to implement a new outpatient service. A plan was developed outlining methods for expanding these services to other parts of the continuum of care at some future date.

In still another community that had a complete mental health and substance abuse continuum of care, the needs assessment discovered that co-occurring disorders treatment services were offered to all subgroups in all parts of the mental health and substance abuse treatment continuums of care except residential treatment and supportive housing. In this instance, individuals in Subgroup IV were excluded from these services by both treatment systems. It was determined that the number of treatment slots currently available for this same subgroup in both outpatient treatment components were not adequate for the number of clients in need of such services. The decision-making process in this instance centered around how to implement co-occurring treatment services in supportive housing and residential treatment settings for individuals with serious mental health and substance abuse symptoms, and how to expand the existing number of outpatient treatment slots. As is true in all instances, new sources of available revenue did not cover the cost of providing all of these new services. The political and professional will in the community supported adequate levels of co-occurring disorders treatment services in all parts of the continuums of care. Enough funding existed to expand outpatient services or add co-occurring disorders treatment services to either residential treatment or supportive housing components, but only one expansion could currently be funded. In this community, the decision was made to incorporate co-occurring disorders treatment services into the residential treatment component. The decision was based on the rationale that it was better to expand the types of services available than to increase the actual number of services; the expanded services should be the most intense type available. A plan was developed to expand outpatient co-occurring disorders treatment services and implement such services into the supportive housing component in the future.

As illustrated previously, the assessment will normally identify more needed services than there are current resources to fund them. Thus, the last step of this process normally involves the development of a fundamental plan in which the community states that its level of service delivery does not adequately meet all the treatment needs of its citizens, and a commitment is made to find ways to provide these services. This plan needs to fully identify all the unmet needs and propose methods and timelines for implementing the needed services. Plans can be a simple paperwork exercise that offers some condolences to the losers in the decision process, or they can truly embody the community's will to implement needed services. Strategies that demonstrate a true commitment to establishing these new services must include the following:

- clear statements of what needs to be implemented;
- methods for implementing these services that can be measured for effectiveness;
- specific timelines for implementation;
- a built-in evaluation process to determine the effectiveness of the strategic plan; and
- a method for modifying the plan should it fail to achieve its objectives.

For example, a plan that identifies the need for new or additional co-occurring disorders treatment services but has little data justifying this need will not be able to withstand competing demands for the same money. Furthermore, a plan that lacks a clear hierarchy of needed services (which services should be implemented next, and so on), demonstrates a lack of community consensus about which services are most needed. This lack of consensus will undermine the possibility for a unified position by the professional and advocate community, and greatly hinder their ability to lobby for the needed funds. If the plan lacks identification of specific methods to obtain the needed resources (such as submitting grants to public or private agencies or examining if Medicaid funds can be used for such services) at the time the plan is written, then it is unlikely that busy program managers will have the time or energy to think of such strategies. The plan must also be constructed with a built-in timeline and a process for evaluating its efficacy and the community's continuing support. A fundamental plan that is not reviewed annually by the stakeholders in the community and modified if necessary is just a piece of paper collecting dust. When decisions are made concerning which new treatment services will be implemented and for which portion of the co-occurring disorders population, there are always immediate winners and losers. One way of ensuring that there are no permanent losers in this process is the continued implementation of the fundamental plan.

CONCLUSION

The heterogeneity of individuals with co-occurring disorders requires that those who implement treatment programs decide which subgroups they are prepared to treat. This decision is based on several factors, including the services needed, current and projected service capacities, staff skill levels, general mission of the program, availability of other community treatment support resources, funding limitations, and the political will of the community. This chapter discussed how to identify the subgroups of this population; how to conduct a comprehensive needs assessment of the community's mental health and substance abuse treatment services; how to decide which services will be offered for which subgroups; and how to develop an effective plan for implementing needed co-occurring disorders treatment services. The next chapter focuses on the issues involved in developing and designing services after the target population and general type of services has been agreed upon.

Chapter 4

Planning for New Co-Occurring Disorders Treatment Services

Once the target population is defined and the general type of services to be provided is agreed to, the next step is to develop a plan for their implementation. Six important decisions must be made during this planning process:

1. Defining which specific treatment services are to be provided.
2. Establishing appropriate client-to-staff ratios and total annual client capacity for these services.
3. Determining who will provide the services and where will they be provided.
4. Deciding when the services will begin.
5. Designating what organizational structure the services will use.
6. Identifying methods for establishing relationships with existing mental health and substance abuse treatment programs and other community agencies that provide essential support services for this target population.

The purpose of this chapter is to examine common issues that arise when attempting to make these decisions during the planning process and present ways that these issues can be successfully resolved.

IDENTIFYING SPECIFIC SERVICES TO BE IMPLEMENTED

Chapter 2 presented seven types of core services that need to be available to clients in each component of the mental health and substance abuse continuums of care to ensure that comprehensive co-occurring disorders treatment services are provided. In some cases a program will only need to add a few of these core services to existing ones to achieve comprehensiveness, while in other cases all of these core services will need to be established in a program. As is often the case with incomplete continuums of care, funding and other limitations may hinder the full implementation of these core services. In those cases, this portion of the planning process must include a method for ensuring how those services will be implemented in the future. Also, other essential support services needed to ensure program effectiveness, such as child care for a women's outpatient co-occurring disorders treatment program will need to be identified. The following scenarios discuss ways the planning process can ensure that new services are comprehensive.

It was decided to add new outpatient co-occurring treatment services for Subgroups II and IV to the services of an existing community mental health center. The center already has access to psychiatric stabilization services, provides medication service, has a psycho-education program on mental illness and medication management, and routinely provides case management services and links clients with other community agencies for additional services. The following services must be added to ensure comprehensiveness:

- the ability to provide detoxification;
- a psychoeducation series on how alcohol and other drug use interacts with mental disorders and another that covers relapse prevention skills;
- integrated individual, group, and family treatment;
- the ability to test for substance use; and
- knowledge of and promotion of participation in mental health and substance use self-help recovery groups.

Once the number and type of services needed are identified, part of the design and planning process must address how they will be implemented. During this particular planning process, the members of the planning committee facilitated a memorandum of understanding (MOU) between the mental health center and the local public detoxification center. The MOU ensured that clients who were not in need of psychiatric hospitalization would be accepted for detoxification services. Another MOU with the existing psychiatric stabilization facility ensured detoxification services would be provided for individuals hospitalized for psychiatric symptoms. The planning process also identified existing psychoeducation curricula concerning the interaction of alcohol, drugs, and mental disorders, as well as substance abuse relapse prevention skills that can be acquired. The plan set aside funds for these curricula and established a method for training staff in their use. Likewise, a training and supervision methodology was developed for staff who provide integrated individual and group therapy interventions. It was also decided that breath and urine testing would be used to monitor substance use and funds were set aside for purchasing the equipment to provide these tests. The mental health center offered space and helped initiate self-help meetings for clients and the community. The center also encouraged the use of the facility for meetings of the local chapter of the alliance for the mentally ill. Finally, it was decided that integrated family treatment service was not possible at this time because neither new nor existing staff had all the necessary skills. Once the new staff becomes proficient at providing integrated individual and group treatment, one staff member will then receive additional family therapy training. When that individual is fully trained, the integrated family therapy modality will be implemented.

At a substance abuse residential treatment program it was decided to add co-occurring disorders treatment services for Subgroup IV. The existing programs already provided or had access to detoxification services, medication services, integrated psychoeducation programs, integrated individual and group counseling services, substance use testing methods, and established methods of linking clients with self-help groups designed for individuals with mental health and substance use disorders for their Subgroup III clients. Still needed was the ability to provide inpatient treatment for individuals who became unstable because of psychiatric symptoms; ensuring that clinical staff had the knowledge and abilities to provide extensive case management services for the new target population; initiating an integrated family therapy modality; and establishing working relationships with local mental health self-help and support organizations.

As in the previous planning scenario, the plan included the need to develop an MOU between the residential treatment facility and the local public program providing psychiatric stabilization services.

The plan also included methods for developing and implementing a training program for staff concerning how to effectively provide case management services for individuals in Subgroup IV. A training program was also included in the plan for increasing the family therapy skills of staff already providing integrated treatment so that modality was available to the residents of this treatment facility. Finally, strategies were identified in the plan for establishing working relationships between the facility and the local mental health advocacy and self-help community.

In another situation, a new agency initiated a supportive housing program for individuals in Subgroups II, III, and IV. In this instance, the supportive housing program was a new service being provided by a new agency and had none of the core co-occurring disorders treatment services in place. The plan had to include methods to ensure that each of these seven core services were provided for residents in the housing program. The need for and strategies for establishing MOUs between these new services and local detoxification and psychiatric stabilization facilities was included in the plan. The plan outlined that medication services, psychoeducation, and integrated treatment continued to be provided by agencies referring clients to these supportive housing services. The plan, however, outlined a training program that required staff working in these new services to be knowledgeable about medication compliance, medication side effects, relapse prevention issues, and the nature of co-occurring disorders treatment. The plan also differentiated which case management responsibilities pertained to referral agencies and which case management responsibilities pertained to staff of the new services. Funds were included in the plan to purchase substance use testing equipment and self-help expectations of the residents were detailed as well as methods for promoting this participation. The goal of this part of the planning process for new co-occurring disorders treatment services was to ensure that the clients received all the necessary core services.

ESTABLISHING CLIENT/STAFF RATIOS AND PROGRAM CAPACITY

All new treatment services must have plans in place to determine how many clients can be treated at any given time and how many can be treated annually. The first figure is based on client/staff ratios and the second figure is based on the average length of time that clients stay in treatment. Client/staff ratios normally reflect the amount of time required to adequately meet the treatment needs of clients. Staff working with individuals who need intensive case management, multiple treatment sessions per week, and who are prone to medical or psychological crises obviously cannot have as many clients on their caseload as staff working with stable individuals who attend treatment once a week and have little or no case management needs. Reis's four-subgroup model described in Chapter 3 can provide guidance in determining staff/client ratios. Subgroups I (low psychiatric and substance use symptoms) and III (high substance abuse and low psychiatric symptoms) tend to need less case management and other labor-intensive interventions. Subgroups II (high psychiatric and low substance use symptoms) and IV (high psychiatric and high substance use symptoms) normally need substantial case management and more intensive treatment interventions. Thus the targeted population for these services will help determine what staff/client ratios will be established. Depending on the nature of the clients being served, the total treatment capacity of an outpatient program will vary depending on the clients' functioning levels. It has been my experience that a caseload of fifteen to twenty is a good benchmark for a full-time therapist working with clients in Subgroups II and IV, and a caseload of twenty-five to thirty is a reasonable benchmark for a full-time therapist working with clients in Subgroups I and III. These ratios are somewhat lower than normal ratios for substance abuse and mental health treatment programs because clients with co-occurring disorders will normally need more attention than clients with just a single disorder.

Once the staff/client ratios are determined, the annual service capacity of a program can be established. As indicated previously, this is accomplished by multiplying the total treatment capacity at any given time by the average turnover rate of each treatment slot. Some clients will drop out of treatment after one day and other clients may stay in treatment for years. The turnover rate is the average length of stay of all these clients. Obviously, new services will not know their actual turnover rates for at least a year, so initial estimates of annual service capacity need to utilize findings from other programs. Hendrickson and Schmal (2000) found that over an eighteen-year period, the average length of stay was seven months for individuals in

Subgroups II and IV during their first treatment admission to an outpatient setting. They also stated that four other outpatient programs treating a similar population, although not reporting average length of stay, did document very similar retention rates through the first year of treatment (Burnam et al., 1995; Case, 1991; Hanson, Kramer, and Gross, 1990; Kofoed et al., 1986). Using the seven-month average length of stay figure, it can be estimated that 1.6 treatment episodes would be provided by each outpatient treatment slot annually. Little research has been conducted concerning average treatment length for these two subgroups in residential settings. Bartels and Thomas (1991) found that the average stay in a six-month residential program was sixty-seven days or approximately two months, and Burnam and colleagues (1995) found that the average stay for a homeless portion of this population in a long-term therapeutic community (TC) that provided treatment for a year or more was 227 days or approximately 7.5 months.

Subgroups I and III are often found in traditional substance abuse treatment programs and thus examination of average lengths of stay in those programs can be used to estimate average lengths of stay for these types of clients. The Drug and Alcohol Services Information System (2002), using the Treatment Episode Data Set (TEDS) of 2,000 of 348,000 substance abuse treatment records submitted by eighteen states, reported that the average stay in outpatient treatment was ninety-three days or approximately three months. It also reported that the average stay of long-term residential programs was sixty-three days or approximately two months.

Planners of new co-occurring disorders treatment programs can use these estimates to determine the annual treatment capacity of the new services being planned. For example, it can be estimated that new outpatient services with three full-time staff providing clinical services to clients in Subgroups II and IV could treat between seventy-two to ninety-six clients per year (1.6 clients × 15 treatment slots × 3 staff = 72 clients per year, or 1.6 clients × 20 treatment slots × 3 staff = 96 clients per year). Likewise it can be estimated that a residential program for Subgroups I and III could treat six clients for each bed that they have (6 clients × 8 beds = 48 clients per year). Of course these are estimates based on very limited research, but they can provide some working estimates that planners can use to determine if the amount of services that they plan to offer will meet the actual demands identified by the community. It will be important that new services maintain records that allow them to determine their actual average lengths of stay so that they will be working with their real numbers in future years. However, this information will not be available to a program for at least a year.

DETERMINING WHO WILL PROVIDE THE SERVICES AND WHERE THEY WILL BE HELD

Once the target population and the type and amount of services to be implemented have been identified, the next step is to determine who will provide the services and where will they be held. This determination is based on several factors, including the following:

- which subgroups compose the target population;
- willingness of existing agencies to provide such services;
- best location for these services;
- availability of essential support services; and
- the general community and professional political atmosphere.

The purpose of this section is to examine these factors and discuss how best to determine who will provide the services and where will they be located.

Traditionally, mental health programs have been designed to treat individuals with serious mental disorders, and substance abuse programs have been designed to treat individuals with serious substance use disorders. Hence, in clinical terms Subgroup III (high substance abuse symptoms and low psychiatric symptoms) would best fit into a substance abuse setting, while Subgroup II (high psychiatric symptoms and low substance use symptoms) would best fit into a mental health setting. Though Subgroup I (low psychiatric and low substance use symptoms) is often found in private practice settings, these individuals will still find their way into public and private nonprofit substance abuse and mental health treatment settings. They may become involved in a substance abuse treatment program because of a driving while intoxicated (DWI) charge, or they may enroll in a mental health treatment program to obtain medication. Clinically, this subgroup could fit into either treatment setting. The setting they end up in is usually dictated more by the reason treatment is being requested than the treatment needs. Likewise, Subgroup IV (high psychiatric symptoms and high substance use symptoms) might be found in either a mental health or substance abuse setting depending on why treatment is sought. Clinically, these individuals best fit into the mental health system because most will continue to need long-term support for their mental disorder after their substance use disorder is in full remission.

Regardless of which treatment setting might make the most sense for a subgroup, the treatment setting must be willing to provide appropriate treatment for that subgroup. A substance abuse treatment program based on the philosophy that the use of medication is not congruent with full recovery would not be able to provide effective treatment for clients in Subgroup III, many of whom need medication. Likewise, a mental health program based on the philosophy of not addressing or taking a position about personal alcohol and drug use could not provide effective treatment services for individuals in Subgroup IV. It is not necessary that all program staff be able to provide effective co-occurring treatment before such services are introduced into that treatment setting (see Chapter 6 concerning staff training and development issues), but it is necessary that the program accept as part of its mission the treatment of a particular subgroup and a willingness to establish those necessary qualities and services outlined in Chapter 2.

These services are best located where the client will receive the bulk of treatment and where treatment is easily accessible. Convenient locations will greatly promote engagement and full participation by clients. Many clients enter co-occurring treatment services under some requirement of the court, social service agencies, or the family, and thus are ambivalent about treatment. Requiring them to receive services at multiple locations or at a location not easily accessible will only increase their resistance and ambivalence toward treatment. In addition, Subgroups II and IV often do not have the means, psychiatric stability, and life skills to travel to multiple treatment sites or get to treatment locations not easily accessible. A program that requires clients to go to one location for their intake/assessment, another location for their psychoeducation series, another location for their individual and group treatment, and still another location to leave urine samples places significant barriers to client engagement and retention for treatment of co-occurring disorders.

Many individuals being treated for co-occurring disorders are in need of additional support services in order to establish and maintain long-term recovery. These support services range from health providers to housing and financial assistance. The more functionally impaired an individual is the more likely additional support will be needed. Subgroups II and IV will normally need multiple support services and a portion of Subgroup III will also need such services. In most instances, substance abuse and mental health treatment programs have developed working relationships with the agencies that provide services their clients often need, such as HIV testing or job training. Likewise most mental health treatment programs work with agencies that provide supportive housing or psychosocial activities. Decisions concerning where to place new services must consider whether the needed supportive services are in place at that program and, if lacking, must determine if the program has the ability to establish such relationships.

Finally, the community and professional political atmosphere plays an important part in determining where these new treatment services will be located. Funding is often directly related to the political support provided by politicians, advocacy groups, and professional organizations. New funds for co-occurring disorders treatment services are much more likely to be provided to programs that are viewed as effective and cooperative. Programs that have had conflict with these political entities in the past are least likely to receive new funding. Decision makers must take this reality into consideration when determining where to place these new treatment services. Obviously some level of conflict will always exist between treatment services and their political supporters; however, the key to any location decision is determining if placing services within a specific program will kill the establishment or effectiveness of these new services. If either case is true then placing these new treatment services in that program should be avoided and an alternative location found.

The decision of where to place these new services must take each of these factors into consideration. In a specific community the local substance abuse treatment program leaders express a desire to expand the program's mission to treat individuals who fall into Subgroup III. Since the program staff is supportive of this and the required changes would be minimal, it is expected that the program can provide effective treatment services for this population. Also such a program would most likely have already developed working relationships with other agencies that provide essential support services for this population. In this instance it would be expected that the political and professional agencies of that community would support location of these new services in the substance abuse treatment program. However, in another situation it might be decided to locate these services in the local mental health program because the substance abuse program staff might believe that introducing medication and flexible lengths of stay into their treatment program would undermine the treatment they provide to other clients. In this situation, the mental health program staff will need to have new treatment practices such as urinalysis introduced into their setting, and establish working relationships with agencies not previously worked with, such as the local detoxification center. Another situation may occur in which neither the mental health nor the substance abuse treatment programs are willing to provide treatment for individuals in Subgroup IV. In that instance it might be decided to establish a new treatment program for that population. This program will then need to establish its own treatment practices, develop relationships with agencies that provide support services for mental health and substance abuse clients, and develop its own political support base. The decision of where to locate treatment services is normally the result of a compromise between what is ideal and what is possible.

DETERMINING WHEN THE SERVICES WILL BEGIN

Determining a start date for services is a complicated process and involves the following:

- developing a realistic time frame for hiring and/or training staff;
- constructing or remodeling existing facilities;
- establishing a functional and clear admission and referral process; and
- developing a marketing strategy of services that will ensure adequate client levels.

It has been my experience that most time frames established by program developers and managers to accomplish these tasks are greatly underestimated and thus most programs begin much later than originally announced.

Underestimates can create three potential problems. The first problem is that staff is hired too long before services are implemented. This very expensive portion of a program's budget is wasted because no services are being provided. Furthermore, this situation can create potential morale or boredom problems for staff that can continue long after services begin. The second potential problem results from the excitement and anticipation that is generated in the professional community when it is announced that a new treatment program is to begin. Even though most experienced professionals in the field are used to programs beginning long after the announced dates, their normal emotional and cognitive response is still "great, another program that overpromises what it can offer." A program that starts later than originally announced will suffer some loss of credibility, and professionals in the community may be hesitant at first to refer clients to its services. The third potential problem is that community advocates who had to use some of their political capital to help create this new service may feel let down by the program's late opening. They may have made promises to clients, family members, oversight organizations, and other significant persons in the community based on dates given them. Such a situation has the potential of lessening the community support that the program will need to survive in the long run.

The bottom line in establishing a start date is that it is always better to begin services earlier than the announced start date rather than later. Thus it is better to overestimate the time it takes to establish new services. To establish a reasonable start date, three factors must be taken into consideration. These are (1) time needed to make the treatment facility ready for services, (2) time required to hire the staff necessary to begin services, and (3) time needed to develop the operational procedures that facilitate client access and flow through the treatment program. These three processes are normally interrelated and occur in a parallel manner; however, each has its own set of barriers that can interfere with its completion.

Most planning bodies for mental health and substance abuse treatment services do not have members with extensive construction experience, which is a primary cause for services opening later than planned. I would highly recommend that planning activities for such new services include an individual with construction management experience by either including this person in the planning (such as a family member whose child will receive these services or a previous client who now does this type of work) or by consulting a professional to determine if the timelines are reasonable.

New services will either move into an existing facility or require a new one. Existing facilities will have either adequate space to handle the new services (a truly rare event), or will have to reconfigure existing space or build an addition. New facilities require that a building be found, remodeled, or built from scratch. Also, both existing and new facilities need the necessary building permits and zoning clearances before services can be offered. When remodeling or doing new construction, at least 25 percent should be added to the time that construction firms estimate it will take to complete the work to cover unexpected work delays for weather or labor problems. Because space reconfiguration normally involves such issues as staff room changes, walls going up or down, personal and public spaces becoming smaller, and changes in access to phone, computer, fax, and copying equipment, most staff members will be negatively affected in some way. Management must give some thought to how the angry and hurt feelings regarding space reconfiguration will be addressed and processed.

Without adequate staff there can be no effective co-occurring disorders treatment services. At a minimum, the new facility needs to have management, supervision, clinical, and administrative support functions in place before providing services. Depending on the size and location of the new services, the number of new staff members that must be in place will vary greatly. If new services are being introduced into an existing program in which management, supervision, and administrative support functions will be provided by existing staff, it is possible that only one of the new clinical positions will need to be filled before beginning services. Depending on clinician availability and the programmatic policies concerning when staff can be hired, the program might be able to provide the human resources needed to begin these services the first day that funding is available. Chapters 6, 7, and 8 provide detailed discussions concerning issues involved in hiring management, supervisory, clinical, and administrative support positions for co-occurring disorders treatment services.

If the services are being initiated in a new stand-alone program, staff providing all four of the previously mentioned functions must be in place before the program can open. In that instance, the position of program manager must be filled first. Then, depending on the program's size, that individual might also provide the clinical supervision and possibly some administrative support functions. In the first instance, the amount of time needed to have essential staff in place will probably be fairly short because clinical staff can be interviewed as soon as the manager/supervisor is hired. However, in the latter instance, first the program manager must be hired. This manager must then hire a clinical supervisor and the head administrator, who in turn must hire clinicians and other administrative support persons. In this case, hiring will be a lengthy process and many months may pass before all positions are filled.

Policies and procedures concerning client admission, treatment practices, and discharge procedures are vital in order to describe the program to referral sources, clinicians providing the services, and clients participating in them. (See Chapter 8 for a detailed discussion of policies and procedures manuals for co-occurring disorders treatment programs.) An operations manual covering these issues must be at least in draft format before services are offered. Ideally, this manual should be developed jointly by individuals providing all four of the essential functions previously mentioned to ensure continuity and consistency. At a minimum, individuals involved in program management and clinical supervision must participate in its development. These sections of the program's policy and procedures manual do not need to be totally complete to begin services; however, they should at least be in final draft form and provide answers to most questions that referral agencies, clinicians, and clients ask about admission, treatment requirements, and reasons for discharge. Time required to develop this manual will be directly proportional to the amount of staff time that can be dedicated to it, and whether the manual is developed from scratch or is being modified from an existing one. Several staff members dedicating substantial work hours toward modifying an existing manual will take much less time than one staff member spending two hours a week developing a completely new manual.

Obviously various parts of the community will exert pressure to move quickly in implementing these services. However, if unrealistic start times are presented to the community or if services are begun before the needed infrastructure is in place the planners' standing in the community will decrease. The planning body must resist the temptation to promise an unrealistic start date, and must be prepared to make the case to the community why a specific amount of time is required before the services can begin. If facility, staff, and policy and procedure issues are given careful consideration during the planning process, then a realistic time frame can be established and justified.

CHOOSING AN ORGANIZATIONAL MODEL

Numerous organizational models are used to provide mental health and substance abuse treatment services. These models range from traditional hierarchical to matrix-collaborative structures. Several key factors must be considered when choosing the organizational model for these new services. First, will the services be established in an existing program? Second, with what organizations will the staff and clients of these services have frequent contact? Third, what will be the temperament and nature of the staff and clients of these new services? When choosing a workable organizational model for these new services, each of these three factors must be thoroughly examined during the planning process.

New treatment services for co-occurring disorders being introduced into an existing program must use an organizational model that is congruent with the existing one. For example, a decision was made to initiate treatment services for clients with high substance abuse symptoms and low psychiatric symptoms (Subgroup III) into a substance abuse treatment program that provides detoxification and residential treatment services. The current organizational model is a combination of a hierarchical model in which decisions concerning program policies and rules are made almost solely by management and transmitted to the staff, and a collaborative team approach in which clinical decisions are made by a process of discussion and consensus building by a team composed of all the clinicians. Because of this, the length of treatment services is prescribed by fairly inflexible timelines. No one is allowed to remain in the detoxification phase of the program for more than fourteen days and no one is allowed to remain in the residential phase of the program for more than 100 days. This policy has been strictly enforced by the management. Individuals with psychiatric symptoms may require longer treatment stays in the detoxification phase in order to be stable enough to enter the residential phase. Individuals with more than one disorder may not be able to complete all the residential treatment requirements in 100 days. One way of modifying the organizational structure of the existing program without completely forcing an intolerable change upon it is to eliminate the cap on the number of days individuals can stay in either phase. The decision can still be made to go beyond the fourteen and 100 days within the purview of the management, based on recommendations and justifications of the clinical team. The management still has the final word; however, the clinical team now has input into discussions concerning length of treatment. Modifying the organizational structure creates the flexibility in treatment length needed by this population, but at the same time continues to allow the final decision to be made at the management level.

Because the staff and clients of these new services will frequently interact with other community organizations, an organizational model must facilitate these interactions. For example, a decision was made to initiate outpatient co-occurring disorders treatment in a private nonprofit agency that provides a psychosocial program for individuals with serious psychiatric symptoms (Subgroups II and IV). This program uses a slightly modified clubhouse model that involves the program's members (clients) in all aspects of its functioning including answering the phone, helping to write one's own case notes, or helping one another obtain assistance from community services. The organization model is egalitarian, with little power distinction between the various functions performed by staff members. Almost all program design and service decisions are made according to majority votes of the members. With such an organizational model, confusion can occur during interactions with other community agencies. It is quite possible that a member might call another agency to help facilitate services for another member; or another agency might call to talk with a member's worker only to be connected directly to that member or a friend of that member. Other service professionals who are not familiar with this organizational model may be uncertain how to respond to these types of interactions and thus services may not be accessed or they may be discontinued. In such a situation it would probably be advisable to modify the organizational model slightly by designating staff to at least initially interact with agencies not familiar or comfortable with this model. Thus if a member needs some form of support services, a staff member could make the initial contact, inquiring if the other agency is willing to deal directly with members. If that agency cannot do so, then the staff member obtains the information necessary to access those services. Such a modification would create a less egalitarian model for interactions with other agencies, but would not significantly change the internal decision-making procedures of the psychosocial program.

Finally, the organizational model must facilitate the type of work environment that best meets the needs of the clients and allows the staff to make effective use of their skills. For example, new treatment services for clients with multiple psychiatric symptoms and either multiple or few substance use symptoms (Subgroups II and IV) will need a treatment environment that is welcoming and flexible. Staff members must be able to create and carry out individualized treatment plans and be able to operate somewhat independently to respond quickly to unexpected crises. The use of a hierarchical organizational model that requires standard treatment for all clients and prior supervisory permission before deviating from the prescribed treatment would be ineffective for such new services. Organizational models that emphasize power sharing, encourage staff independence and creative work, or advocate teams that share the same work would be more effective with these subgroups.

The final decision concerning which organizational model to use for new co-occurring disorders services will always be the product of the push and pull between these three factors. For example, a decision was made that the organizational model to be initiated in an outpatient substance abuse treatment program for Subgroups I and III will be a mixture of a hierarchical management, matrix-clinical supervision, and democratic team-based treatment. This decision is made because it is perceived that substantial resistance exists to these new services among the current program's clinical staff. Using the existing hierarchical management approach can be useful in sending a clear message to existing staff that these services will be introduced and adjustments must be made. The matrix-clinical supervision and team-based treatment structures are chosen because the new services will be the product of integrating new staff with mental health treatment skills with existing staff that have substance abuse treatment skills. The purpose of this integration is to cross-train all staff in the treatment of co-occurring disorders. It is planned that all staff will eventually be able to treat clients with and without co-occurring disorders. To accomplish this cross-training, conjoint supervision will be provided by two clinical supervisors. One will have mental health treatment expertise and one will have substance abuse treatment expertise (see Chapter 7 concerning issues of joint supervision). The democratic treatment team model recognizes all staff as having equal expertise and acts as a peer cross-training vehicle. The planning process must also consider that the initial organizational model may serve the purpose for only a limited time. In the previous example, once co-occurring treatment services are fully in place and the staff is cross-trained, it will no longer be necessary to maintain matrix-clinical supervision and hierarchical management may no longer best meet the needs of the program. The planning process must therefore recommend a means of reevaluating the organizational model on a regular basis.

IDENTIFYING ESSENTIAL RELATIONSHIPS WITH OTHER COMMUNITY AGENCIES

Treatment services for individuals with co-occurring disorders never occur in a vacuum. The very nature of these disorders causes numerous negative impacts in many individuals' life spheres. Individuals with co-occurring disorders will often have a wide variety of health problems, need substantial support in resolving financial and housing difficulties, or need assistance in obtaining and maintaining employment. At a minimum, working relationships will need to be established with agencies that provide health, financial aid, housing, and employment services. Many other support services may also be needed depending on the nature of the identified target population such as child care, transportation, or parent skill training. Because of this, planning activities for new treatment services must identify essential support services that these clients will also need. This process must not only identify the needed services, but also who in the community provides them and how relationships will be developed with these service providers. Figure 4.1 provides a tool that planning groups can use or modify to identify needed support services and community agencies that provide them. Chapter 8 discusses in detail

Service Category	Provider Agency	Client-Provider Relationship
Financial		
Housing		
Medical		
etc.		

FIGURE 4.1. Sample Form for Tracking Existing Community Support Services

methods of developing and maintaining relationships with agencies that provide essential support services.

CONCLUSION

This chapter focused on developing a plan for implementing treatment services once the target population is identified. This plan involves the following:

- determining what services will be offered;
- establishing staff/client ratios;
- deciding where these services will be held and who will provide them;
- deciding when the services will begin;
- choosing an organizational model; and
- identifying other community agencies with which to establish working relationships.

The development of this plan is a fluid process that is impacted by many competing forces. It is essential that at the start of the planning process it be acknowledged that compromises will have to be made. The key, or the art, of effective compromising is determining which compromises will make the program ineffective and which ones will only cause inconveniences. Obviously the former will require firm stands by the planning group, and the latter will require the group to be flexible. Two important questions to ask when attempting to decide either to stand firm or compromise are: "Will this compromise eliminate services essential to achieving the goals of abstinence and psychiatric stability?" or, "Will this compromise create barriers which make access to services too difficult for the target population?" I believe a yes answer to either of these questions will result in ineffective services and thus a compromise should not be made. In all other instances everything is negotiable. The next chapter addresses the many issues that can arise when these services are actually implemented.

Chapter 5

Implementing a New Treatment Service

Once a co-occurring disorders target population has been identified and a plan developed for providing appropriate treatment services, the next step is to implement these services. The implementation phase of new services usually covers the first two years of of the service, during which many adjustments may be made to the original design. Adjustments made tend to result from the setting into which the new treatment services are placed. In almost all instances, the following new treatment services will be established in one of four types of service settings:

- an existing mental health treatment program
- an existing substance abuse treatment program
- a new setting just for the treatment of co-occurring disorders
- a setting whose primary purpose is neither the provision of mental health nor substance abuse treatment (such as a welfare-to-work social service program or a correctional institute)

Regardless of the setting, new co-occurring disorders treatment services will require changes in the culture of existing settings or the development of new ones. This chapter will examine common issues that arise when co-occurring disorders treatment services are initiated in each of these four settings and provide suggestions concerning ways these issues can be effectively addressed.

IMPLEMENTATION IN AN EXISTING TREATMENT SETTING

The introduction of co-occurring disorders treatment services into an existing mental health treatment setting results in multiple conflicts and learning opportunities for the staff, clinical supervisors, and managers of such programs. Minkoff (1993) identified eight flash points in which potential conflict can occur between mental health and substance abuse practices. These include the following:

- peer counseling versus medical/professional treatment models;
- spiritual recovery versus scientific recovery;
- self-help versus medication;
- confrontation and expectation versus individualized support and flexibility;
- detachment/empowerment versus case management/care;
- episodic treatment versus continuity of responsibility;
- recovery ideology versus deinstitutionalization ideology; and
- psychopathology secondary to addiction versus substance use secondary to psychopathology.

Lee (1982) identified five areas in which social workers and alcoholism counselors differ in their treatment approaches.

1. Social workers are nondirective; alcoholism counselors are directive.
2. Social workers attempt crisis reduction; alcoholism counselors attempt to orchestrate a crisis.
3. Social workers attempt to reduce stress; alcoholism counselors attempt to increase stress.
4. Social workers wait for clients to identify problem areas; alcoholism counselors work toward defining the problem with observations.
5. Social workers look for the underlying cause of the drinking; alcoholism counselors believe alcohol is the cause.

Minkoff (1993) also identified fifteen parallels or similarities concerning the treatment of substance use and major mental disorders as follows:

Both are biological illnesses.
Both are hereditary in part.
Both are chronic.
Both are incurable.
Both lead to lack of control of behavior and emotions.

Both have positive and negative symptoms.
Both affect the whole family.
The disease progresses in the absence of treatment.
Both have symptoms that can be controlled with proper treatment.
Both have denial of the illness.
Both often lead to depression and despair.
Both are often regarded as moral issues resulting from personal weakness rather than biological causes.
Guilt and failure are often felt.
Shame and stigma are experienced.
The illnesses are in part physical, mental, and spiritual.

The push and pull between these similarities and differences is the genesis of most of the issues faced by existing mental health and substance abuse programs when co-occurring disorders treatment is introduced into their settings.

Mental Health Settings

Treatment philosophy, treatment practices, and relationships with other community organizations are issues that arise when services for co-occurring disorders are introduced into a mental health center.

Treatment Philosophy

Treatment philosophy includes the following questions:

Are substance use disorders biologically based?
Should the goal of treatment be abstinence?
Should clients be required to address issues that they do not want to address?

Treatment Practices

Common treatment issues result from the following:

• being more confrontational concerning differences between what a client says and does

- using psychoeducation and group treatment more extensively than individual treatment
- using more directive interventions
- increasing use of self-disclosure
- asking clients to provide urine, breath, or hair samples to determine current alcohol or other drug use

Relationships with Community Organizations

Relationships with community organizations include the following issues:

> increased contact with the courts and other agencies of the criminal justice system, such as sending reports about the client's progress and participation
>
> developing effective relationships with agencies not worked with before that provide essential support services to the program's clients
>
> increased referral of clients to self-help groups (Alcoholics Anonymous, Narcotics Anonymous, Al-Anon, or SMART-Rational Recovery)

Chapter 6 outlines specific knowledge and skills that mental health professionals must understand to be effective in treating individuals with co-occurring disorders.

In general but not always, when treatment for co-occurring disorders is introduced into an existing mental health setting, the target population will be individuals with significant psychiatric symptoms (Subgroups II and IV). The staff is most familiar with these subgroups and the agency normally has many of the necessary support services already in place.

Implementation Decisions

Three major decisions were made during the design phase concerning implementation of services. The first decision concerned who will work with this population. Will all staff provide co-occurring treatment services? Will some staff provide these services while others do not, or will all staff provide some limited services while certain designated staff provide the comprehensive services? The second decision concerned delivery of services. Will individual, case management, group, or family modalities be used? How often will they be used and for what purpose? How long will the services last? What will be the general purpose of these services? The third decision concerned location of the services within the facility. Will the services be placed throughout the agency or will the services be held in only one part of the facility? The answers to these questions greatly influence which issues arise when the new services are implemented.

Outpatient Services

New outpatient treatment services for co-occurring disorders were implemented into an existing outpatient community mental health center. It was decided that one existing and several new staff members will specialize in the treatment of co-occurring disorders. All clients falling into Subgroup IV (high psychiatric and substance use symptoms) will have one of these specialists assigned as their therapist, as will some clients falling into Subgroup II (high psychiatric symptoms and low substance use symptoms). Depending on staff availability, Subgroup II individuals might be assigned a therapist who does not specialize in treating co-occurring disorders, but these clients will be able to participate in all group treatment services for such disorders. All services for co-occurring disorders will be held in one section of the mental health facility.

Changes in Treatment Philosophy and Practice

In this particular instance issues arose regarding changes in treatment philosophy and practices. Some clients were now forced to address issues (primarily substance abuse) that they did not regard as problematic, and some changes in treatment practices included therapists using much more directive interventions and testing for drug use. These changes generated a great deal of tension between the existing mental health therapists and the new therapists for co-occurring disorders. The mental health therapists believed that clients should be able to choose issues to work on. They also believed that drug testing is degrading, violates clients' privacy, and interferes with the therapeutic relationship. The co-occurring disorders therapists believed the new philosophy and treatment practices were essential if these clients were to achieve abstinence and psychiatric stability and believed the mental health staff to be naive about how powerful substance use disorders are. There was also limited contact between the two staffs because the services for co-occurring disorders were held in a separate section of the building. Because of these differences, the agency's mental health therapists were hesitant to refer existing or new clients to these new services. This created a problem for the agency: The census of the new treatment services remained low and many clients in need of such services did not receive them.

Staff Interaction

The agency decided to address this issue by creating more interaction between the two staffs focusing on increasing both personal contact and the exchange of ideas. To promote more personal contact between the two staffs, treatment services for co-occurring disorders and the offices of the staff providing these services were spread throughout the building. The staff for co-occurring disorders, while still maintaining its own specialized supervision, began to participate periodically in other supervision groups for the purpose of discussing cases suspected of substance use. A presentation to all mental health staff was provided by the unit for co-occurring disorders concerning services provided, practices used, and how to formally refer or informally discuss clients who could benefit from these services. It was hoped that this increased would generate trust, resulting in a greater likelihood that clients in need of such treatment services will be referred.

Implementation Within a Hospital Setting

New treatment services for co-occurring disorders were implemented into a short-term psychiatric stabilization inpatient (hospital) setting. Because all clients were experiencing a psychiatric emergency, they fell into Subgroups II and IV (high psychiatric symptoms and either high or low substance use symptoms). It was decided that two staff members would provide specialized services. Clients in need of such services might have any staff member as a primary worker because clients were randomly assigned the next available clinician as their primary worker at the time of admission. All specialized treatment services were to be held in one group room of the facility.

In this instance the issues centered on treatment practices and relationships with other community agencies. Detoxification, though always provided when needed, was never an acknowledged part of the mission of this facility until the introduction of the new treatment services for co-occurring disorders. A greater number of individuals who needed detoxification were admitted to the facility due to the introduction of these new services. This required all staff to become more competent in identifying and dealing with withdrawal symptoms and becoming more sophisticated in dealing with substance use disorders in genral. As identification increased it soon became apparent that the vast majority of clients admitted to this facility had co-occurring disorders and that having just two staff members designated to deal with such clients was insufficient. In addition, community agencies began to refer more individuals with less severe psychiatric symptoms who needed detoxification. This resulted in either accepting inappropriate clients, spending significant amounts of time connecting these clients with more appropriate services, or turning them away.

The facility staff decided to address these internal and external issues in several ways. First they decided to formally train all current clinicians in identifying and addressing co-occurring disorders. Second, all future staff vacancies were filled only with individuals already cross-trained or who had the ability and desire to acquire such skills. Once the training was completed, all staff were designated as specialists for co-occurring disorders, and clients were no longer placed in separate groups. Instead, all groups incorporated co-occurring disorders issues into the existing topic of discussion. To address inappropriate referrals, the facility first developed a dialogue with the agencies that most often made inappropriate referrals. This dialogue increased an agency's understanding of the admission criteria for this facility. A point of contact was also established for each agency to discuss the appropriateness of a particular client for the facility. Once these measures were in place, the facility began to enforce its admission criteria. When a client referred by one of these agencies was not admitted the staff member designated as the point of contact called to explain why a client did not meet the admission criteria. By making all staff members treatment specialists for co-occurring disorders, the facility better reflected the population it was actually treating. By establishing a dialogue with specific community agencies, the facility increased the potential to reduce the number of inappropriate referrals.

Implementation Within a Group Home

New treatment services for co-occurring disorders were implemented into a twelve-bed group home for individuals with serious mental disorders. Some of the residents had co-occurring disorders and some did not. Those that did fell into Subgroups II and IV (high psychiatric symptoms and either high or low substance use symptoms). Because all staff would have contact with all residents at some time, all staff members would need the ability to address these co-occurring disorders. The head counselor had a master's degree, while the remaining staff had either bachelors degrees or were not degreed. Treatment services for co-occurring disorders included individual and case management services, two weekly treatment groups, and transportation to local self-help groups. As this was a residential facility, the co-occurring treatment services were provided throughout the facility.

The issues that arose in this situation centered on treatment philosophy and practices. Although it was expected that all staff would provide the treatment services, it soon became apparent that some staff members simply lacked the education or temperament to be effective with these clients. Salary limitations made it difficult to hire more qualified staff. Because previous residents with alcohol and other drug use issues had been excluded from the group home, the staff did not have experience in dealing with use issues. Soon after the first individuals with co-occurring disorders were admitted to the group home, incidents began to occur concerning substance use in the home or clients returning to the group home intoxicated. Staff reactions to these incidents split along three viewpoints. Some staff believed any use should result in immediate removal from the group home; some staff believed the residents should be able to drink as long as they are not disruptive; and other staff believed that all clients should be abstinent, but each incident should be addressed individually. This situation resulted in residents receiving mixed messages from the staff concerning substance use, as well as inconsistent interventions. Much chaos ensued, including conflicts between staff members, conflicts between residents and staff members, and ineffective treatment for co-occurring disorders.

The executive director of the agency that manages this group home appointed a work group composed of group home staff representing each viewpoint, the lead counselor, the staff member at the main agency's office who oversees this and other group homes, and two professionals from the community who have experience in co-occurring disorders treatment. The goal of the group was to examine issues and develop group home policies for the agency concerning substance use. The agency also hired a consultant to facilitate the discussion of the work group. After much discussion, comment, and voicing of disagreements, the work group proposed a policy that required abstinence by all group home residents and outlined a process for addressing violations of this rule, allowing each incident to be individually evaluated. Consequences could range from none to removal from the facility. The executive director endorsed the proposal and made the oversight manager and the lead counselor jointly responsible for implementing it. Only certain group home staff could address treatment issues for co-occurring disorders. The remaining staff directed any identified co-occurring disorders treatment issues to the staff providing those services. Sending a consistent message to the clients concerning substance use and having the most capable staff provide the services resulted in increased quality service and the group home provided both a sober and safe living environment.

Implementation Within an Assertive Community Treatment Team

In still another instance, new treatment services for co-occurring disorders were implemented into an Assertive Community Treatment Team (ACT Team). This was accomplished by adding a treatment specialist for co-occurring disorders to the team. The ACT model involves taking all the services needed by individuals with serious mental disorders directly to them in the community rather than just providing these services at the mental health center. Thus it is hoped that clients who will not or cannot participate in treatment at a facility would still be able to remain stable in the community. Each member of the team had a specialty such as nursing, case management, employment, housing, and so forth; however, all were equally responsible for all the services that clients on the team needed. Clients placed on the ACT Team were unable or unwilling to participate in normal outpatient mental health treatment activities. They stayed on the team until they no longer needed its services. Clients seen by this team were in Subgroups II and IV (high psychiatric symptoms and either high or low substance use symptoms). The treatment services took place wherever ACT Team services occurred (at the client's home, at the ACT Team's office, on the street, etc.).

The issues that arose from the implementation of these new treatment services for co-occurring disorders centered on treatment philosophy and practices. Simply placing a specialist for co-occurring treatment disorders on the team did not increase the skills of other team members in dealing with substance use disorders, nor did it modify any of the existing practices of the team. Because the new staff member was but one individual on the team and needed to fit in, this person began to lose professional identity and avoided practices that could cause conflicts with other team members. As a result, substance use issues were not being addressed any more significantly than before this position was added. Because substance use greatly increases the risk of hospitalization for individuals with serious mental disorders, hospitalization rates for ACT Team clients were much higher than would normally be expected. Questions began to arise concerning the cost effectiveness of this team.

Originally, the management of the mental health agency was aware of the relationship between substance use and hospitalization, so they had added the specialist for co-occurring disorders to the team. Alarmed by the continued hospitalization rate, they examined factors contributing to hospitalizations. It was found that no reduction occurred in the number of ACT Team clients for whom substance use played an important part in their hospitalizations. This resulted in the establishment of a management work group that examined the substance use treatment practices of the ACT Team. The work group concluded that substance use was not vigorously addressed by the team and that the new specialist did not have supervisory support to introduce substance use philosophies or practices. As a result of these findings, it was written in the team leader's performance standards that it was his or her duty to ensure that all clients were continually assessed for substance use and that those found with substance use disorders would have treatment goals and objectives concerning those behaviors included in their treatment plans. Quarterly reviews documented how these goals and objectives were addressed. The substance use behaviors of each client also became part of regular supervisory case reviews. To reinforce the professional identity of the specialist, the specialist was to play an active advisory role both for the team leader and the other team members in the development of their treatment roles. This ensured that substance use issues were addressed by state-of-the-art practices. Also, to more fully reinforce professional identity, it was arranged for the specialist to become part of a substance abuse supervisory group run by the agency's substance abuse supervisor. All ACT Team members would also attend at least one co-occurring disorder treatment training session during the following year. The management of the agency hoped by increasing the awareness and skills of the ACT Team's members concerning co-occurring disorders and significantly increasing the voice of the team's co-occurring disorders specialist in the development of treatment plans, that the team would more vigorously address substance use disorders.

Substance Abuse Settings

As is true when treatment services for co-occurring disorders are added to a mental health treatment setting, implementing such services into existing substance abuse treatment settings also brings new and often alien practices to that program. The difference is that these new practices and values come from the mental health field. Also as previously discussed, the issues that these new values and practices generate center on treatment philosophy, treatment practices, and relationships with other community organizations. Changes in treatment philosophy may include not initially requiring abstinence, terminating clients so that they can hit bottom, or being less demanding and structured about requirements from clients. Treatment practice changes may include using more individual and case management interventions; promoting medication use; not requiring self-help attendance until a client is able to attend; or being less directive. Changes in relationships may include developing working relationships with psychiatric hospitals and crisis intervention programs, or learning about and developing relationships with agencies that provide essential support services such as housing, finance, health, or employment.

In general but not always, when co-occurring disorders treatment is introduced into an existing substance abuse setting, the target population will likely be individuals with less significant psychiatric symptoms and either significant or less significant substance use symptoms (Subgroups I and III). As in mental health settings, the issues that arise will be determined by the decisions made during the design phase such as who will provide the service, the structure of the services, and where services will be located. The following are examples of common issues that arise and how they might be successfully addressed.

Residential Treatment Programs

Ten new treatment beds for individuals with co-occurring disorders were introduced into an existing ninety-day substance abuse residential treatment program. The new clients had high substance use symptoms and low psychiatric symptoms (Subgroup III) and had been in Subgroup IV (high psychiatric and substance use symptoms) but who now were psychiatrically stable. Two staff members from the existing program were transferred into the new co-occurring disorders unit and two additional new staff members were hired to provide the treatment services. It was decided that a special track be established for clients with co-occurring disorders and that all their services, except for self-help activities, be held in a separate area of the facility.

The issues that arose from the implementation of these new treatment services centered on treatment philosophy and practices. One of the transferred staff members questioned some of the mental health diagnoses of some clients, particularly those whose symptoms were not severe or were well controlled by medication. This staff member believed these symptoms may have resulted from long-term withdrawal effects or character defects and thus questioned the use of medication for these individuals. Another clinical issue centered on the relationship between the staff and the psychiatrist. Were they equals on a treatment team or does the psychiatrist have the final say about treatment? A great deal of anxiety was experienced by two of the clinicians when individuals with serious mental disorders began to exhibit elevated symptoms. In one instance, elevated symptoms resulted in a client being detained and hospitalized, resulting in increased anxiety and tension on the unit. Also, it soon became apparent that many clients needed more than ninety days of residential treatment, and aftercare placement in treatment, housing, and employment required much more case management time than the agency had been accustomed to providing. These issues created some tension and anxiety between staff members that was subsequently transmitted to the clients, thus making the atmosphere of the program nontherapeutic at times. Also, clients were discharged before they were ready and sometimes did not have the necessary community supports in place resulting in significant relapse that necessitated return for residential treatment.

The management of the program became aware that treatment success rates for this population were ineffective and hired a consultant to evaluate these services. The consultant identified the previously mentioned problems and made the following suggestions: (1) the staff member who questioned the existence of certain mental disorders should be transferred back to non-co-occurring disorders services and be replaced with a therapist who is interested in working with this population; (2) all co-occurring disorders staff should receive intensive training in dealing with psychiatric symptoms and monitoring medication compliance and side effects; (3) length of stay should be individualized and graduation be based on moving through levels of treatment instead of length of treatment; and (4) staff time should be reallocated so that the new levels of case management are taken into consideration. The management accepted and implemented these recommendations. Management also made it quite clear through the supervisory process that although each professional in the program has a specific function, all are equal members on a treatment team. These modifications helped to increase the stability experienced by clients in the treatment program and increased the chances of long-term recovery once clients were discharged from the program.

Outpatient Treatment Programs

An outpatient substance abuse treatment program that was already treating individuals with lower psychiatric symptoms and either higher or lower substance use symptoms (Subgroups I and III) added treatment services for individuals in Subgroups II and IV (higher psychiatric symptoms and either lower or higher substance use symptoms). Prior to the addition of these services all staff had been expected to treat Subgroups I and III and had integrated them into their caseloads. It was decided to have only two staff members provide the case management and therapy services for these new clients, with the existing psychoeducation series about the effects of alcohol and other drugs open to their clients. No maximum or minimum length of treatment was required and the existing psychiatrist and psychologist provided medication and psychological testing services. No special place in the facility was dedicated exclusively to the services of these new clients.

Although it would appear that the addition of these clients would go smoothly because the staff and program are already used to treating co-occurring disorders, issues still arose concerning treatment practices and relationships with community agencies. The intake workers at times had difficulty determining who should be assigned to regular therapists and who should be assigned to the two new therapists. This resulted in some clients being transferred between therapists after starting treatment. It was soon apparent that some of the new clients were disruptive in the program's psychoeducational groups or did not seem to benefit from them. No procedures were in place to deal with psychiatric emergencies on site, so when they occurred it created a great deal of chaos in the treatment facility. The agency also had no established relationships with agencies that provided essential support services to these individuals, such as psychosocial activities, supportive employment, or supportive housing, thus resulting in a great deal of case management time being spent identifying and connecting clients with those services. Finally, the other agencies in the community had discovered these new services and the demand soon exceeded the treatment resources of the program. These issues resulted in increased time between initial appointment and connection with appropriate treatment services, reduction in time available for direct treatment services, and the establishment of a treatment waiting list.

To address these issues the program's management established a work group composed of the intake workers and the new clinicians. The group devised clear placement guidelines for new clients with higher psychiatric symptoms. A procedure was initiated to discuss clients who fall into gray areas between subgroups before they are assigned a therapist. Specific psychoeducation groups were created for these clients rather than mainstreaming them. Procedures were also established to deal with psychiatric emergencies and a working relationship was established with the agency providing these services in the community. Memorandums of understandings (MOUs) were established with community agencies providing services for individuals with serious mental disorders. The MOUs designated specific referral procedures and obligations to provide services, which decreased the case management time needed to access these services. Finally, a treatment enhancement grant was submitted to fund additional treatment positions for this population. Until those funds were received, an additional staff member was designated to treat these clients and thus shorten the waiting list. These actions had the potential to increase the speed with which these clients would receive appropriate services, to ensure that their special needs were met in all aspects of their treatment, and to reduce the time dedicated to connecting these clients with appropriate support services.

Outpatient Opiate Replacement Program

In another instance, new co-occurring disorders treatment services were added to an outpatient opiate replacement program. The clients fell into Subgroup III (higher substance use symptoms and lower psychiatric symptoms) and Subgroup IV (higher psychiatric and substance use symptoms). In addition to attending daily treatment for opiate replacement and other related activities, they also attended three specialized co-occurring disorders treatment groups per week. All individuals with co-occurring disorders were assigned one of two therapists who had been designated to work with this population. The physician providing the opiate replacement also provided their psychiatric medication. They received co-occurring disorders treatment within all parts of the treatment facility.

The issues that arose from the implementation of these new treatment services centered on treatment philosophy and practices and relationships with community agencies. Those implementing the program soon discovered that individuals in Subgroup IV were very different from individuals in Subgroup III. Individuals in Subgroup III had little difficulty following the program rules, fitting in with other clients, and getting to the program on time for opiate replacement. Individuals in Subgroup IV experienced psychiatric symptoms that at times interfered with their ability to successfully implement the program. At times program managers had difficulty deciding if the cause of these behaviors were psychiatric or resulted from willful disregard of the program's rules. Because of these differences, it also soon became apparent that these two subgroups did not work well together in the same treatment segment. Also, no procedure was in place for continuing opiate replacement therapy when an individual was hospitalized for psychiatric symptoms. The program managers had little experience working with agencies that provided community support services for individuals with serious mental disorders. These issues resulted in the following: clients missed their daily opiate replacement; some clients were discharged prematurely, and some clients were retained who should have been discharged; an ineffective treatment group for those with co-occurring disorders; and some clients did not receive essential support services.

After examining these issues, the program's management decided that individuals in Subgroup III could easily be absorbed into the regular caseloads and services of the program. This would require minimal staff training regarding the nature of these psychiatric disorders and medication issues. Those individuals in Subgroup IV were in as much need of intensive case management as they were in need of regular treatment, so the designated therapists were initially assigned to work with this population only. This reduced their caseload sizes and allowed them to develop essential relationships and procedures for connecting these individuals to support services in the community. It also allowed them to provide a daily treatment group just for individuals in this subgroup. If necessary, outreach help was provided to transport individuals to the clinic for opiate replacement therapy if they were having difficulty getting there. An agreement was also signed with the local psychiatric hospital that allowed clients to continue their opiate replacement therapy should they be hospitalized. These actions increased the chances that all individuals with co-occurring disorders would receive the level of services they needed, while not being disruptive to the services other clients were receiving.

Nonmedical Detoxification Program

In still another instance, co-occurring disorders treatment services were added to a nonmedical seven- to ten-day detoxification program. These services were targeted for individuals in Subgroups III and IV (higher substance use symptoms and either higher or lower psychiatric symptoms) who need neither medical nor psychiatric hospitalization. All medical, nursing, and clinical staff members were expected to work with these individuals; however, one clinician was assigned as the primary worker for all individuals with co-occurring disorders. These individuals participated in all activities of the detoxification center and also attended a specialized psychoeducation group three days per week run by the clinician. This structure resulted in co-occurring treatment services taking place in all parts of the detoxification facility.

The issues that arose from the implementation of these new treatment services centered on treatment philosophy and practices. A primary issue concerned distinguishing between substance-induced symptoms and true co-occurring disorders. Since all clients in a detoxification phase experience some level of depression and anxiety, there arose a great debate among staff members about who had a co-occurring disorder and who did not. This debate also centered on who should be medicated and when medication should occur. Also related to this debate was distinguishing between a psychotic disorder exacerbated by the stress of withdrawal or the onset of delirium tremens (DTs). The staff had a wide range of training, education, skills, and experience which greatly influenced the various positions they took. As a result, clients received inconsistent treatment interventions and were given mixed messages concerning their diagnosis and need for medication. Also, the nature of service delivery caused the primary therapist who was to address clients' special needs to spend less time with them than other staff members spent.

To address these issues, the program's management decided that a clearer diagnostic procedure needed to be implemented, and a stronger leadership system needed to be in place to ensure that internal staff debate did not result in inconsistent treatment interventions. To accomplish this, an outside consultant who specialized in diagnosing co-occurring disorders was hired to review current diagnostic procedures and make recommendations concerning how they should be modified. Once this was completed, the consultant also provided training for all staff on the new procedures and the rationale behind them. The program manager was to communicate to staff, and enforce when necessary, that staff members were to stay within their training and function boundaries when working with individuals diagnosed with co-occurring disorders. The diagnosis established by the center's psychiatrist was to guide all treatment interventions, though of course the diagnosis could be modified from information provided by staff observations. It was further communicated that all co-occurring disorders treatment issues would be addressed by the primary staff member assigned to these clients; that when clients mentioned these issues they were to be directed to discuss them with their particular therapist. By taking these actions the management increased the chances that clients would receive clear messages concerning their diagnosis and treatment needs. Treatment for co-occurring disorders provided by the designated staff member was strengthened.

IMPLEMENTATION IN A STAND-ALONE PROGRAM

When treatment services for co-occurring disorders are initiated in a stand-alone program it usually means that neither the substance abuse nor the mental health treatment programs in the community have a commitment to treat the target population. A stand-alone program must develop a completely new culture from which to operate. This evolving culture will have its roots both in the mental health and substance abuse treatment fields. Professionals from both fields will usually compose the staff of new programs. Because new staff will bring with them the values and traditions of their training and treatment experience, all the treatment philosophy and practices and community agency issues found in existing mental health and substance abuse treatment programs may surface when new stand-alone treatment services are implemented. However, this scenario is different because no established ways of functioning exist, and all new staff entering the program are on a more or less equal footing. Any or all of the four subgroups might be targeted for these services. The following are examples of common issues that arise and how they might be successfully addressed.

Residential Stand-Alone Program

A new twelve-bed residential treatment program was initiated for individuals in Subgroup IV (higher psychiatric symptoms and higher substance use symptoms). The new program was initiated because the existing substance abuse residential treatment program could not integrate these individuals into its treatment facility. Individual and group treatments were provided daily and a family program was held on the weekend. A great deal of case management was also provided by the staff. No time limit was determined for treatment; however, it was expected that most individuals would complete treatment within six months. As is the case for all examples in this section, all staff members were dedicated to treating co-occurring disorders and all parts of the facility were dedicated to these services.

Implementation Issues

The issues that arose from the implementation of these new co-occurring treatment services centered on treatment philosophy and practices and relationships with community agencies. Four staff members had been hired for the program; two had previously worked primarily in substance abuse residential settings and two had worked primarily in mental health group homes. The staff with substance abuse treatment backgrounds believed that more confrontation was needed concerning the clients' substance use history; the staff with the mental health background believed that the clients needed very gentle interventions. A great deal of debate occurred between staff members concerning the efficacy of group treatment compared to individual treatment, with the substance abuse background staff taking the group position and the mental health background staff taking the individual treatment position. Also, it soon became apparent that most clients were not ready to return to outpatient treatment within six months and that many who returned to outpatient treatment relapsed in a short time. These issues resulted in general tension among staff members that was transmitted at times to the clients. These issues also resulted in inconsistent treatment interventions, a longer than anticipated waiting list and time period to access these services, and an emerging community view that these high-cost-per-client services were not effective.

Residential treatment work is normally very intensive and this was especially true in this program for individuals with higher substance use and mental health symptoms. This level of intensity often facilitates very strong working alliances among staff members so that no one feels alone with all the therapeutic issues that continually barrage them. Thus, to address the philosophical issues the program's management decided to divide the staff into two teams, each team treating six clients. Each team had one staff member with a mental health background and one member with a substance abuse background, and each team received separate supervision. The purpose was to break up the natural alliances that had formed based on common treatment backgrounds, and thus force the staff to begin blending their treatment approaches needed to form the necessary working alliance. This process was then reinforced during the supervision. More effective working relationships were needed with the outpatient programs that provided the aftercare services for these clients. Therefore, a reentry phase was put in place. During this phase, clients nearing completion of treatment would participate in some of the outpatient treatment services forty-five days to two months before their discharge. Also, more attention was given to connecting the clients to residential settings that had substantial support services. These actions increased the chances that staff would naturally begin to blend substance abuse and mental health approaches into integrated intervention practices, would better prepare clients for their transition to outpatient treatment, and would provide them with the needed residential support to live on their own, thus improving long-term treatment outcomes.

Stand-Alone Outpatient Program

A new co-occurring disorders outpatient program was initiated for any individual with both a substance use disorder and mental disorder (all four subgroups). The new program was established because neither the mental health nor the substance abuse outpatient treatment programs had been able to provide effective services for these individuals. The services provided by four outpatient therapists used the individual, case management, group, and family treatment modalities. Individuals who had higher psychiatric symptoms (Subgroups II and IV) were placed in one treatment track; individuals with lower psychiatric symptoms (Subgroups I and III) were placed in another treatment track. As with the previous case, no time limit was set on treatment; however, it was expected that few individuals would remain in treatment for more than nine months to one year.

Implementation Issues

The issues that arose from the implementation of these new treatment services for clients with co-occurring disorders centered on treatment practices and relationships with community agencies. The biggest issue that arose after the implementation of these services was the lack of a full continuum of care for this population. The outpatient treatment services staff soon found themselves attempting to treat individuals who were more in need of detoxification services or residential treatment than outpatient treatment. These clients periodically absorbed a great deal of the therapists' time, though few positive outcomes resulted from these efforts. Furthermore, these clients often had a negative impact on the progress of other clients, either by being disruptive in treatment groups or by encouraging other clients to use alcohol or other drugs or actually giving them these substances. A greater number of clients than expected left the program early and treatment outcomes were much lower than expected. As these issues became common knowledge in the community, other community support services which normally provided services for these individuals became more selective or resistant to accepting them into services. This created a great deal of frustration among the program's clinical staff that resulted in a high staff turnover rate, further disrupting clients' services.

The program management's primary strategy to address these issues centered on limiting their services only to clients who were appropriate for outpatient treatment. To accomplish this, management worked with the clinicians who developed very clear admission criteria that excluded clients who would most likely not achieve abstinence on an outpatient basis. Strategy also included a process for discharging clients who disrupted the program's treatment activities. This was a difficult choice for the program's management and the clinicians to make and enforce. Obviously individuals who were not admitted were in need of treatment, so it was difficult to deny them services. However, by taking this position the program's staff provided the appropriate level of treatment to the clients who were admitted, which resulted in longer stays and better treatment outcomes. This also eventually resulted in easier access to the community agencies providing support services to the program's clients, and staff turnover stabilized. Though the program initially received substantial flack from the community for denying treatment services to certain individuals, the staff worked hard to communicate the clinical reasons behind these decisions. They also attempted to form alliances with community advocacy groups to promote co-occurring disorders treatment services in detoxification and residential settings. Ultimately these actions increased the chances that all individuals with co-occurring disorders would receive the appropriate level of care.

Stand-Alone Multipurpose Agency

In another instance, a new agency for those with co-occurring disorders was developed that provided outpatient, residential, psychosocial treatment and supportive housing for individuals with higher psychiatric symptoms and lower or higher substance use symptoms (Subgroups II and IV). The new services were developed because neither the substance use nor the mental health programs providing these services could work with these clients. It was decided that the four modalities of individual, case management, group, and family would be used by each component of the new program. A client could initially enter treatment in any of the agency's treatment components and could then move back and forth between all treatment components, depending on their service needs. No time limits were placed on any service component or on how long a client could receive services from the agency.

Implementation Issues

Though these services sound like a truly seamless system, issues arose regarding treatment philosophy and practices and relationships with community agencies. Though the services were provided by one agency, each component was in a separate location with different staffs and different supervisors. The supervisors met regularly with one another but the staff did not. This resulted in staff being more identified with their component than with the agency as a whole. Each component also began to develop its own treatment philosophy and ways of handling clinical issues. For example, the residential program required attendance at all group sessions; however, the psychosocial component clients could choose to attend or not. Each component also began to develop working relationships with agencies that frequently referred clients to them or provided support services frequently used by clients in that phase of treatment. For example, the outpatient component developed strong working relationships with local substance abuse and mental health treatment programs that frequently referred clients. This group also worked with the community agency that provided supportive employment services for these clients. The residential treatment component formed a strong working relationship with the local detoxification program that frequently referred clients to this component, and also with the local community agency that provided health and financial assistance for these clients. All this resulted in clients receiving inconsistent treatment messages. Relationships were established between the agency's components and community agencies, but not between these community agencies and the agency itself. Problems arose that the agency did not realize, as well as the establishment of territoriality and tensions between the agency's components. In general, the agency began to operate as four separate programs instead of one.

The agency's management decided to address these issues by strengthening its case management services. The case management function was removed from each component and a separate case management unit was created whose supervisor became part of the agency's senior management team. All clients were assigned a case manager when first admitted to the agency's treatment services, and this case manager remained their primary worker, regardless of which treatment component they participated in. This case manager was responsible for coordinating all internal treatment activities and connecting the client with essential community support services. The agency also began to hold monthly staff meetings for all agency staff members. Meetings focused both on administrative and clinical issues, but also facilitated more interaction between the different components' staffs. The agency also established a rotation system for new staff members so they would spend the first month of their employment observing and participating in the services of all the agency's components. Also, when appropriate, staff members were encouraged to apply for and fill vacancies in other parts of the agency. These actions had the potential to increase staff interactions; increase the staff's view that they were working for an agency instead of a component; increase consistent treatment interventions; and increase unified procedures for working with referral agencies or accessing support services for the agency's clients.

Stand-Alone Crisis Program

In another instance, a new co-occurring disorders program was established for individuals with co-occurring disorders who are in a crisis as the result of their psychiatric and substance use symptoms. Treatment services offered by the program include crisis assessment and intervention, a thirty-bed crisis stabilization and detoxification facility, and aftercare placement case management services. Treatment services were targeted for Subgroups II, III, and IV (clients with higher psychiatric symptoms or substance use symptoms or both). Crisis intervention, individual and group treatment, family support and reintegration, and case management services were offered. Nonmedical detoxification was used; individuals in need of medical detoxification were referred to the local hospital. It was expected that most individuals presenting for services would receive a single service and then be reconnected to their existing community outpatient services or have an initial intake arranged. It was also expected that individuals admitted to the detoxification and crisis stabilization facility would stay in that facility on average for seven to ten days and then be referred to residential or outpatient treatment. No distinction was made between psychiatric and detoxification beds because it was expected that the majority of clients would need both services. It was also expected that all staff would be able to address both mental health and substance abuse issues.

Implementation Issues

The issues that arose from the implementation of these new treatment services centered on treatment philosophy and practices and relationships with community agencies. The first difficulty this program experienced was differentiating between co-occurring disorders and a single substance use or mental disorder. The vast majority of individuals seen had symptoms of both, so questions arose about whether the clients were receiving appropriate treatment services at their outpatient program or whether they should be referred to another facility. A second issue involved staff training: almost all staff members of the new facility had mental health treatment backgrounds, so substance use issues were not as thoroughly examined and addressed and most clients were referred to a mental health facility for aftercare services. The third issue that arose was how to handle clients who kept reappearing for crisis and stabilization services but did not follow through with aftercare services. These issues resulted in clients being referred to treatment facilities that did not fully meet their treatment needs. Referrals to mental health facilities resulting in longer waits for intakes, and a significant number of clients returned frequently for crisis services but quickly became unstable again, causing disruptions for their families and the community.

The management team of the crisis center decided to address these issues in several ways. First, they brought a substance abuse consultant into the agency to increase the substance abuse assessment and treatment skills of the staff. It was also decided to fill vacancies with staff members who had either a co-occurring disorders or a substance abuse treatment background. The team also arranged to hold a joint meeting with all the community agencies it interacted with. The purpose of this meeting was to discuss the assessment issues it experiences and develop liaison relationships with each of these agencies that would allow discussions of the appropriateness of particular referrals. Finally, a decision was made to create a mechanism for identifying clients who use only crisis intervention and stabilization services, and then limit their services to just those which ensure their safety. It was hoped that by limiting services, these clients might be willing to participate in more appropriate long-term services. They also planned to develop working relationships with the families of these clients with the goal of providing the necessary support to families so that they limit all but the essential support to their family member. Here again it is hoped that increasing the client's discomfort will prompt the client to accept additional treatment services. These actions increase the potential that the crisis program will address substance abuse issues in a more comprehensive manner, that clients will be better linked with appropriate aftercare services, and that there will be a reduction in the number of clients who only use crisis stabilization services.

IMPLEMENTATION IN A NON–MENTAL HEALTH OR NON–SUBSTANCE ABUSE SETTING

When co-occurring disorders treatment services are introduced into a non–mental health or non–substance abuse treatment setting it is usually the result of the need to co-locate these services at that location or because such services are not available through the mental health or substance abuse treatment system. When these co-occurring disorders services are established, they are often part of mental health or substance use services being established at that location, though at times only these specialized services are established. When these services are introduced into these agencies, it means that both substance abuse and mental health practices and values are being introduced into a setting whose mission has never been to provide these types of treatment services. These nontraditional treatment settings might include a welfare-to-work social service program, a correctional institute, a homeless shelter, or an employment assistance program. In such instances not only will potential conflicts arise between mental health and substance abuse values and practices, but also between these values and practices and those held by the nontraditional treatment agency. Another important dynamic in these cases that adds to issues that arise when these services are implemented is that these services are often provided by nonstaff from another agency, so the providers must always remember they are guests, not part of the staff of that agency. As in the case of the stand-alone programs it is quite possible that these nontraditional agencies will have clients who fall into any of the four co-occurring disorders subgroups. The following are examples of common issues that arise and how they might be successfully addressed.

Welfare-to-Work Program

Co-occurring disorders treatment services were introduced into a welfare-to-work program. The services are targeted for individuals with mental health and substance use disorders, which include individuals with co-occurring disorders participating in a welfare-to-work social service program. Because these individuals were not following through with referrals to existing treatment services, it was decided to use a portion of the program's funding to create outpatient treatment services on-site. A cross-trained therapist was hired by the agency to provide outpatient treatment for any participant who was identified as having a mental health or a substance use disorder or both. These treatment services are provided as long as the individual is receiving other welfare-to-work services. Services are to be provided using individual and group treatment modalities and are provided on-site where the clients are receiving their other services.

Implementation Issues

The issues that arose from the implementation of these new co-occurring disorders treatment services centered on treatment philosophy and practices and relationships with community agencies. Though the new welfare-to-work philosophy had moved agency practices from providing entitlements to creating expectations, most staff had not yet made the needed emotional shift to be effective with these new practices. Thus when the new therapist proposed attaching treatment attendance to the receipt of benefits many of the agency's staff greatly resisted those efforts. Also the use of urine testing to monitor substance use was considered by many agency staff members as degrading and controlling and thus mixed messages were sent to clients regarding providing urine samples. It was soon determined that a significant number of clients were also in need of psychiatric medication evaluation. Such services were available through the local community mental health center; however, the staff was also ambivalent about requiring such assessments and taking of prescribed medications. Though many of the welfare-to-work staff had some human service training, few fully understood how therapy worked. Thus they often had unrealistic expectations concerning how fast it takes a client to make significant changes. They believed the clients should decide what they wanted to work on and should not be confronted about certain behaviors because it would damage the therapeutic relationship. They had some mythical views about the therapist's ability to know what is going on with clients at all times, being able to logically talk them into something they don't want to do. Conflict also arose over the free exchange of information between the therapist and other staff. The welfare-work staff was used to freely exchanging information about clients with one another. They felt that the therapist was arbitrarily withholding information when they were told that a release of information was needed before client information could be shared. An article by Jacobi, Hendrickson, and Wallace (2002) outlines these and other specific issues that may arise when implementing substance abuse treatment services within a welfare-to-work agency setting. All this resulted in clients receiving inconsistent messages about the need to participate in treatment, and a great deal of tension arose between the therapist and other staff members. Clients often failed to come to initial assessment meetings or attend treatment on a regular basis. Few if any consequences occurred when a client failed to show for treatment services. The therapist therefore felt isolated and misunderstood and indicated to her supervisor that she was very frustrated and was considering looking for a new job. In essence, clients in need of substance abuse and mental health treatment in the welfare-to-work program were not receiving such services.

Addressing the Issues

The agency's management decided to address these issues by contacting the management of the local community mental health center and requesting its help. The agency assigned one of its staff members who was skilled at supervising staff who work with individuals with co-occurring disorders. The staff member consulted with the therapist and the management of the welfare-to-work program. The first decision resulting from this consultation was that the therapist would begin receiving clinical supervision at the community mental health center while still receiving administrative supervision through her current supervisor. The supervisor also began to attend management team meetings of the welfare-to-work agency so that she could have an understanding of the intraworkings and needs of that agency. A training program was designed for the welfare-to-work staff that focused on such topics as confidentiality laws, the nature of therapy, the importance of medication and urine testing, and the importance of leverage in substance abuse treatment. After the training, another consultant was brought in to facilitate several discussions concerning pertinent issues. Such actions increased the potential for the following:

- welfare-to-work staff to be more active in the promotion of client participation in mental health and substance abuse treatment;
- client participation in treatment and regularity of attendance;
- the therapist to receive the clinical supervision needed to help her maintain her professional identity and lessen the need to look elsewhere for work;

- the therapist to develop personal relationships among the community mental health center staff; and
- a better understanding by the therapist of procedures that facilitate client referral for such services as medication.

All these changes would also create better welfare-to-work outcomes.

Correctional Facility

In another instance, co-occurring disorders treatment services were established in a correctional facility that already had a traditional substance abuse unit run by the local public substance abuse treatment program. The new unit services were designed for individuals who had higher substance abuse symptoms and lower psychiatric symptoms (Subgroup III). A private nonprofit agency provided the services with special state funds. A twelve-bed cell block was set aside in which the co-occurring disorders treatment was provided; only individuals with such disorders were placed in the cell block. The treatment model used was a modified therapeutic community with group treatment being the primary modality. Two staff members provided clinical services five days a week and on the weekend the inmates ran their own groups. Guards were present on the cell block at all times. A case manager interviewed potential candidates to determine if they were appropriate for the program and helped to identify aftercare placements for the program's graduates. Individuals must have at least four months remaining on their sentence at the time of admission. It was expected to take about four months for inmates to complete all treatment levels. Some inmates were released to the community when they graduated; other graduates were returned to the correctional institution's general population until they were released.

Implementation Issues

The issues that arose from the implementation of these new co-occurring disorders treatment services centered on treatment philosophy and practices and relationships with community agencies. One issue evolved from the assignment of guards to the treatment unit.

Guards were randomly assigned to all the cell blocks on a weekly basis. This resulted in different guards constantly rotating through the unit. Some guards were supportive of the services and some were not. The unsupportive guards often restricted the treatment activities on the unit under the guise of security concerns, especially on the weekends when the treatment staff was not present. This created a great deal of tension between the treatment staff and some of the guards. Another issue that arose was that some individuals who were more psychiatrically impaired than they first appeared to be were occasionally admitted to the unit. This resulted in considerable chaos for the unit. The correctional institute resisted removing these individuals from the unit and placing them back into the general population because the institution lacked adequate psychiatric resources. The lack of adequate psychiatric resources also resulted in difficulty in getting some clients the medications they needed. An underlying tension existed between the traditional substance abuse program and the new unit. Why, they wondered, did the private program get the funding for the new unit, and did certain clients on the co-occurring disorders unit really have mental disorders? Since the public program provided all the outpatient and residential treatment in the community, questions concerning the continued use of medications and other treatment needs often arose when aftercare plans were made for graduates of the new unit. These issues resulted in rancorous relationships among the three involved staffs, disrupted treatment in the unit, and potentially inadequate treatment following release from the correctional facility.

Addressing the Issues

Since guard interference issues were also experienced by the traditional substance abuse treatment unit, the management of the three organizations met and developed the following plan. The correctional facility agreed to make two changes. The first was to identify which guards were supportive of the unit's treatment activities and to arrange for them to work on the unit whenever possible. When new guards were hired they were given brief training about the purpose and activities of the new unit and were also given an opportunity to volunteer to work in that cell block. Second, the correctional center also agreed to develop a contract with the local mental health center that would increase the availability of psychiatric medication services and provide psychiatric evaluations and behavioral plans for inmates experiencing severe psychiatric symptoms. The treatment program managers agreed to have their staffs participate in a two-day training session provided by correctional facility staff. This training outlined the specific security measures and the reasons behind them that the facility was required to follow. Included in the training was an opportunity to discuss how certain treatment activities could be structured in such a manner that they were congruent with required security measures. In addition, it was agreed that all new staff hired for these treatment programs would go through the same orientation as the new correctional facility staff.

The management of the private provider of the co-occurring disorders treatment and the public substance abuse treatment program also met for the purpose of developing a process to address their philosophical and diagnostic differences. The outcome of this meeting resulted in the development of a training program for both staffs that covered the assessment, diagnosis, and treatment of co-occurring disorders. The training helped staff determine which clients were most appropriate for the programs of each agency, and emphasized that the programs have more similarities than differences.

It was also decided that the two staffs should begin meeting regularly in order to get to know one another and discuss the types of clients each deal with. At this meeting the co-occurring disorders program case manager will bring assessments of potential clients for the new unit so that both staffs can discuss that client's appropriateness. Discharge plans for the unit's clients also began to be developed at the meeting, using input from the public program's staff who had insight into which clients would do best in their various outpatient and residential services. The public substance abuse treatment agency also agreed to initially accept for thirty days the diagnosis and treatment recommendations for clients coming from the co-occurring disorders unit to their outpatient or residential treatment services. At the end of thirty days the client diagnosis and treatment plans would be reassessed. Taking such actions increased the potential for the following:

- client services in the correctional facility will not be disrupted because of nonsupportive staff;

- clients with co-occurring disorders will receive the medication they need;
- the correctional facility will have a process in place to handle individuals with severe psychiatric symptoms;
- clients will not be required to make major changes in their treatment activities until they are well known by the staff of new treatment services; and
- the staffs of both treatment programs could develop a more cooperative and supportive working relationship.

Homeless Shelter and Outreach Center

In another instance, co-occurring disorders treatment services were established in a homeless shelter and outreach center. These services were targeted for anyone with co-occurring disorders who was served by this facility. The outreach staff made contact with homeless individuals in the community and encouraged them to make use of the shelter and other services. The shelter's rules required individuals to leave after sixty days, and after individuals were discharged they could not be readmitted to the shelter for ninety days. These new services were part of a cooperative project between the local mental health and substance abuse treatment agencies that were designed to bring mental health and substance abuse treatment to the clients of this facility. The services were funded by a three-year federal grant. Two therapists were located full time in the facility to provide these services. One worked for the mental health agency and one worked for the substance abuse agency. The mental health therapist worked with individuals who had higher psychiatric symptoms and either lower or higher substance use symptoms (Subgroups II and IV) and the substance abuse therapist worked with individuals who had lower psychiatric symptoms and either higher or lower substance use symptoms (Subgroups I and III). Treatment services included assessments, individual and group interventions, and connecting clients with appropriate treatment once their homelessness was resolved. Services were provided in whatever space was available at the time in the facility.

Implementation Issues

The issues that arose from the implementation of these new co-occurring disorders treatment services centered on treatment philosophy and practices. It is often difficult to initially determine which subgroup a client fell into, therefore, some individuals with less severe psychiatric symptoms ended up with the mental health therapist and some individuals with higher psychiatric symptoms ended up with the substance abuse therapist. Because individuals with differing levels of psychiatric symptoms tend not to function well together in treatment groups (Hendrickson, Schmal, and Ekleberry, 2004), the interactions in the treatment groups were disrupted or a client was required to change therapists in the middle of treatment. Another issue arose between the outreach staff and the two therapists.

The outreach staff believed that these therapists should take their services to the clients currently living on the street, while the therapists believed that these services would be of little use to individuals who were still committed to homelessness. Tension also developed between the shelter staff and the therapists regarding client discharges. The therapists believed that a stay of sixty days was insufficient for many of their clients because their treatment needs were long term and residential treatment and supportive housing slots were limited in the community. Also, the substance abuse therapist questioned whether a single relapse should result in immediate discharge from the shelter. The mental health therapist questioned whether a significant increase in psychiatric symptoms should result in immediate discharge. The shelter staff firmly believed that any substance use should result in discharge and believed they were ill-equipped to handle clients with significant psychiatric symptoms. Disagreement also existed between these two factions concerning the ninety-day wait for readmission to the shelter. These issues resulted in decreased treatment effectiveness; reduced level of cooperation between the staff members of the homeless program and the therapists; and significant numbers of individuals with co-occurring disorders remaining homeless in the community.

Addressing the Issues

The management of the homeless program, the mental health program, and the substance abuse program met and decided to address these issues in several ways. First, they developed a joint policy that clearly stated that the mental health and substance abuse services provided by the therapists be conducted only at the shelter. However, these therapists were now to attend the weekly case review meetings of the outreach staff to provide suggestions concerning how the mental health and substance abuse needs of individuals still living on the street might be addressed and actions the outreach staff might take that would promote action regarding these issues. Second, all treatment groups were to be co-led by both therapists. Hence, both therapists would have treatment contact with all clients and if a client needed to be reassigned between these two therapists minimum disruption would occur in the therapeutic relationship. The third action involved length of stay and readmission requirements. Length of stay for these clients would now be based on their treatment participation and aftercare plan. A client targeted for residential treatment or supportive group housing could remain in the shelter until admitted to those services. Clients who were planning to return to the community and live on their own could remain in the shelter beyond sixty days if it appeared that they were working on their mental health and substance abuse issues. Also, readmission criteria were now based more on individuals' feelings about what they had learned regarding their behaviors that caused homelessness, and plans they had for learning how to manage these behaviors, than on length of time since last admission. The final action was that the mental health program's psychiatric crisis service agreed to evaluate clients who experienced significant increases in their psychiatric symptoms and provide the shelter staff with an intervention and monitoring plan for that client. Discharge then only occurred for threatening or violent behavior, which also might result in hospitalization. Since the crisis services were available twenty-four hours a day and therapists would come to the shelter to perform these evaluations, most shelter staff began to feel more comfortable having individuals with higher levels of psychiatric symptoms in their facility.

It was decided to continue the policy that any substance use would still result in a discharge; however, it was arranged with the substance abuse program's detoxification services that these clients would be accepted into that program, and after a brief stay they could apply for readmission to the shelter. These changes resulted in the following improvements:

- greatly increased the potential for clinical consistency;
- increased cooperative relationships between the staff of all three agencies;

- more accurately addressed housing and treatment needs of these clients; and
- decreased the number of individuals with co-occurring disorders who were homeless in the community.

Free Health Services Clinic

Co-occurring disorders treatment services were established in a free clinic that provided health services to low-income individuals who had no medical insurance. The services were targeted for anyone who had co-occurring disorders (all four subgroups) and were part of the introduction of mental health and substance use services into this clinic. The services were provided by existing staff of the local mental health and substance use programs who had been detailed to the clinic to provide these services. The clinic was open for four hours, four evenings a week, with one mental health and substance abuse therapist there each evening. Two different mental health therapists and two different substance abuse therapists provided these services. Services included assessment, referral, limited brief on-site counseling, and consultation to the medical staff. A private office was available to each therapist, although some of the assessments and interventions took place where other medical services were being provided.

Implementation Issues

The issues that arose from the implementation of these new co-occurring disorders treatment services centered on treatment philosophy and practices and relationships with community agencies. The first issue that arose was the lack of continuity between the mental health, the substance abuse, and the medical staff. Except for rotating doctors, the same medical staff were there each evening; however, this was not true for the mental health and substance abuse staff. This greatly reduced the ability of the staff to develop effective working relationships. No clarity existed concerning which therapist should see clients with co-occurring disorders. The mental health and substance abuse therapist were able to do fairly comprehensive assessments of clients with these treatment needs; however, it soon became apparent that few of the clients identified as needing these services followed through with referrals. Also, several issues arose between the therapists and the medical staff. The first had to do with the therapists having limited knowledge concerning medical conditions and procedures, which created some questions in the minds of the medical staff concerning the therapists' level of competency. The second involved the medical staff, and particularly the doctors, seeing the therapists' primary role as case managers and giving them directives concerning the clients' treatment. The third issue had to do with the medical staff realistically seeing the physical danger these clients were in if they did not address their substance use and psychiatric issues and consequently becoming anxious. This resulted in staff pressuring the therapists to do more than was realistically possible in connecting these individuals with treatment. These issues resulted in limited staff cohesion between the three staffs involved. Thus, few mental health and substance abuse services were used by the clients of the free clinic, other than assessment.

Addressing the Issues

The management of the three agencies involved met and decided to address these issues in the following manner. A single mental health and a single substance abuse therapist would be assigned to the clinic. Thus all three staffs, except for the doctors, would be consistent each evening. The mental health and substance abuse therapists also were to begin attending the staff meetings of the free clinic. In essence these actions were to make the two therapists part of the free clinic's staff.

It was also decided that mental health and substance abuse therapists would begin operating as a team. They would provide joint assessments of each client and then determine afterward to which treatment setting the client should be referred. Also, the therapists were given training regarding common medical conditions found among individuals with mental health and substance use disorders and what the appropriate treatment procedures were for these conditions. In addition, one of the clinic's staff was assigned to be a consultant about medical conditions and their treatment for the therapists.

It was also decided to introduce a psychoeducation program concerning mental health and substance abuse issues that identified clients must attend in order to receive additional services at the clinic. This program was jointly facilitated by the two therapists. Also, non-life-threatening conditions might not receive additional attention at the clinic until the clients entered treatment for their mental health and substance abuse issues. An in-house training was also held concerning the role and functions of these two therapists, which helped to clarify their responsibilities. These management actions resulted in the following improvements:

- increased the potential that the three staffs could develop cohesive and effective working relationships;
- that clients with co-occurring disorders would receive comprehensive assessments and be referred to the appropriate treatment agency;
- that staff from the three agencies would develop a better understanding of what each did and what each was capable of; and
- that clients with mental health and substance abuse treatment needs would become more knowledgeable about these conditions and would enter treatment for them.

CONCLUSION

This chapter focused on the issues that evolve when co-occurring disorders treatment services are implemented in a wide range of agency settings. The specific issues that arise often depend on the type of setting into which the services are introduced. There is no one right way to address these issues; however, flexible approaches usually result in solutions that are beneficial to both the program and the clients. A central theme for all these issues is that all the staff and programs must make changes in the way they work or conduct their business when co-occurring disorders treatment services are introduced into a setting. A full year, and sometimes longer, is needed for staff, management, and clients to adjust to these changes, but it is rare that adjustment does not occur. The next section of this book deals with the many issues involved in the day-to-day management of co-occurring disorders treatment services.

Section III:
Making It Work—
The Day-to-Day Management
of Treatment Services
for Co-Occurring Disorders

Once treatment services for individuals with co-occurring disorders have been established, the spotlight turns to the day-to-day basis of making them work. The first three chapters of this section focus on the human resources issues faced by these treatment services. Chapter 6 outlines the critical issues involved in hiring and training direct service staff. Chapter 7 examines what is involved in effective clinical supervision of these services, and Chapter 8 discusses the tasks involved in effective program management. Chapter 9 focuses on the manner in which these services operate within a larger multilevel/ multi-organizational system, and Chapter 10 describes activities that programs must successfully accomplish if they are to prosper and endure. The purpose of this section is to examine these day-to-day activities that ensure treatment effectiveness and program survival.

Chapter 6

Hiring and Training Clinical Staff

The quality of treatment services for individuals with co-occurring disorders is directly related to the quality of the staff providing these services. Staff hired to provide these services must have or obtain the necessary attitudes, knowledge, and skills needed to provide high-quality services to this population. This chapter reviews the essential knowledge and skill bases that staff must have; describes the types of staff attitudes and temperaments that are most effective with this population; makes recommendations concerning how the application, interviewing, and hiring process can be most effectively used to identify applicants with these qualities; and because most staff will not initially have all the necessary skills, knowledge, and attitudes, presents methods of developing, implementing, and evaluating training programs to increase staff competencies.

ESSENTIAL KNOWLEDGE AND SKILLS

In most instances, staff of new co-occurring treatment services will not have all the essential skills, knowledge, and attitudes in their therapeutic repertoire. They often bring either a set of substance abuse or mental health treatment competencies. Table 6.1 outlines the additional knowledge and skills that mental health and substance abuse trained therapists need to add to their therapeutic toolbox to be effective with this population.

Staff members with mental health training and experience backgrounds normally need to learn about the different types of drugs that their clients are using and what short- and long-term effects the drugs may have on their clients. They need to learn how to monitor urine screens or administer breath tests in a manner that does not interfere with the therapeutic relationship. In addition, they must come to un-

TABLE 6.1. Additional Knowledge and Skill Needs

Mental Health Therapists	Substance Abuse Therapists
Nature and effects of psychoactive drugs and the importance of drug testing	Nature and effects of mental disorders
Nature of addiction	Importance of functioning level
Importance of abstinence	Importance of medication
Importance of self-help involvement	Long-term view of self-help involvement
Working with court-referred clients	Engaging self-referred clients
Being more concrete, directive, and confrontive	Being less directive, more flexible, and confronting more gently
Use of self-disclosure	Maintaining clear boundaries

derstand the power and the nature of addiction and not be surprised or offended when clients say they want to abstain but then surrender to cravings and compulsions. Staff members with substance abuse training and experience, on the other hand, need to learn how to identify the various mental disorders that cluster frequently with substance use, and gain an appreciation of how these disorders affect a person's social skills and ability to function independently in the community.

The therapists with substance abuse backgrounds also need to be familiar with the different types of medications used to treat these disorders and be able to identify their side effects. They also must learn how to promote medication compliance and deal with any negative values or attitudes that clients, members of their families, self-help groups, or other substance abuse professionals may have concerning the use of medications. The therapists with the mental health background will need to gain an understanding of the importance of abstinence from alcohol and other drugs for individuals with mental disorders. They will need to learn about the purpose, culture, and traditions of twelve-step self-help groups such as Alcoholics Anonymous and Narcotics Anonymous, and become comfortable promoting clients' participation in these groups. The therapists with substance abuse backgrounds must learn that for some individuals, such as those who have social phobias or paranoid thoughts, attendance at these meetings may need to be a long-term goal instead of one required early in treatment. Therapists will first need to help clients manage their fears about attending such meetings, and teach them what is appropriate to talk about, depending on the type of meeting they are attending. Some meetings may be open to discussion of psychiatric symptoms and others may not. With so many different types of self-help recovery groups now available for both substance use and mental health disorders, both types of therapists need to understand the principles of each in order to help clients select the type of group that is most effective for them.

The therapists with substance abuse backgrounds who are normally used to having court-ordered clients must learn how to engage self-referred clients, or individuals with whom the court has little leverage. Therapists with mental health backgrounds must learn to work with clients whose only perceived problem is getting the court system off their backs. Thus substance abuse therapists must learn to be less directive, more flexible, and gentler during confrontations in an effort to engage and keep clients who are not court ordered. Mental health therapists, meanwhile, must learn to be more concrete and directive in setting treatment contracts. They need to learn to use psychoeducation and confrontational feedback techniques to motivate some clients to address their substance use. Such techniques also may help these clients in controlling some of their psychiatric symptoms.

The therapist whose professional mental health training may have taught him or her never to self-disclose must learn that some clients need self-disclosure to help them differentiate normal feelings and behaviors from those generated by their mental health or substance use disorders. For example, a client who had just ended a significant relationship was experiencing a significant increase in depressive symptoms and attributed this to her medication no longer working. The mental health therapist can assure the client by telling her that's exactly how she or her friends felt when ending such a relationship; such feelings are normal and will pass with time. The therapist with the substance abuse training background, on the other hand, must learn that maintaining clear boundaries is essential when interacting with some clients. Substance abuse therapists, especially if they themselves are recovering, are used to sharing with clients the history of dependency, and may in fact encounter clients when attending self-help meetings. However, for clients with certain psychotic, anxiety, and personality disorders, too much self-disclosure or even a simple touch of a shoulder can trigger confusion concerning what is intended or really meant. Thus substance abuse therapists must learn to be much more withholding with certain clients than they have been in the past.

Finally, both mental health and substance abuse therapists must learn that words they use in their everyday work may have very different meanings for professionals in another field. For example, when a therapist with training in mental health uses the term "defense mechanisms," she means a psychological process that protects individuals from pain and thus helps them function effectively in the community. The therapist with training in substance abuse, of course, sees defense mechanisms as a negative process that prevents clients from recognizing and acknowledging that they have a substance use disorder. When a therapist with a substance abuse background uses the term "enabling," he is referring to a behavior that protects individuals from the consequences of their substance use and thus contributes to continued use. The therapist with a mental health background may see enabling as a positive process that is often used in behavioral training or case management services to promote effective community functioning, such as helping a client learn how to ride the bus or go to a job interview. Similarly, a therapist with a mental health background normally uses the term "residential" to refer to a facility that provides housing and support for individuals but to a substance abuse therapist, the term refers to a form of intensive substance abuse treatment. Both therapists need to learn the multiple definitions for many commonly used psychological terms in order to communicate effectively with each other and avoid misunderstandings.

ESSENTIAL TEMPERAMENTS AND PHILOSOPHY

In addition to having certain knowledge and skills, therapists working with individuals with co-occurring disorders must also possess characteristics of flexibility, optimism, creativity, respectfulness, and cooperativeness if they are to be effective with this population. Staff with these temperaments can treat each client individually, promote optimism about treatment outcome, develop creative treatment interventions, be respectful of the difficulties some clients have making changes, and have the ability to work closely with other professionals serving their clients. The TAUT-SOAR Model (Hendrickson and Schmal, 1993) can be a useful philosophical model for staff working with individuals with co-occurring disorders (see Figure 6.1). This model is based on the premise that the more difficult the clinical issues, the more growth opportunities there are for the therapist.

TAUT stands for Thoughts of incompetence; Apprehension; Unclear what and how to treat; and Treatment avoidance. These are thoughts, feelings, and behaviors that therapists may experience or demonstrate when encountering problems that they believe they are unequipped to treat effectively. For example, the substance abuse therapist might have these reactions to a young adult male client who presents with a history of alcohol and cocaine dependence but also reports hearing voices occasionally and believes that the FBI is following him with helicopters and has bugged his home and car. The mental health therapist might react with TAUT in treating a young female with a history of bipolar disorder who reports drinking excessively and smoking marijuana on a daily basis. When therapists' anxious thoughts and feelings combine with their confusion concerning a treatment approach, the temptation is to avoid treating the client. They may either refer the client to another agency based on the excuse that the client has a principlal diagnosis that they are not mandated to treat, or make treatment demands that a client cannot achieve. The first method, if successful, simply results in either the mental health therapist treating the substance abuse therapist's client or the substance abuse therapist treating the mental health therapist's client, leaving both therapists still feeling capable only of treating

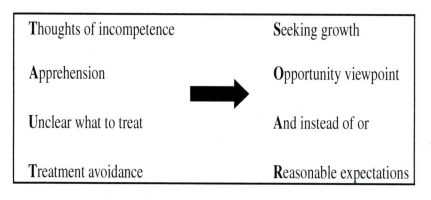

Thoughts of incompetence	Seeking growth
Apprehension	Opportunity viewpoint
Unclear what to treat	And instead of or
Treatment avoidance	Reasonable expectations

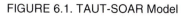

FIGURE 6.1. TAUT-SOAR Model

part of the client's problem. The second method, such as the mental health therapist requiring her client to stop all alcohol and drug use before offering medication or other services, or the substance abuse therapist requiring his very paranoid client to attend ninety Alcoholics Anonymous meetings in ninety days, inevitably leads to clients dropping out of treatment. The therapist has achieved his or her goal not to treat the individual, but the client remains untreated.

To engage and maintain such clients in treatment, both the substance abuse and the mental health therapist must approach treatment from a different perspective. The second part of our model, SOAR, stands for **S**eeks growth, **O**pportunity viewpoint, "**A**nd" instead of "or", and **R**easonable expectations. This approach allows therapists to view their clients with less anxiety, more optimism, and more flexibility. Treating these clients becomes an opportunity for the therapists to expand their knowledge about mental disorders and treatment techniques. The client often presents with a history of many treatment failures, so the therapist can feel free to try various techniques with hopes of finding one that works. Each client becomes a research project with an opportunity for that client to obtain something he or she had not yet achieved—a treatment success. Furthermore, therapists never have to forget what they already know; however, they now have the opportunity to expand that knowledge and integrate the new and old knowledge into a broader paradigm, which ultimately makes them more effective.

Finally, once a therapist decides to treat an individual with co-occurring disorders, he or she can establish more reasonable expectations. For example, the mental health therapist can help a client attend an alcohol and drug education class as a first step in addressing the substance abuse disorders; the substance abuse therapist may introduce the concept of schizophrenia to the client, and slowly move him or her toward a medication evaluation while probing to understand how the psychiatric symptoms impact the client's substance use. Approaching treatment from a SOAR viewpoint increases the chances that the client will remain in treatment and helps therapists gain confidence in their ability to promote change in clients who have complex problems.

THE APPLICATION, INTERVIEWING, AND HIRING DECISION PROCESS

The front door for any program's acquisition of human resources is the application, interviewing, and hiring decision process. Since hiring decisions are always based on limited amounts of information, it is important that the application and interviewing components of this process yield as much information as possible about potential employees. This section describes key pieces of information that should be obtained on the application form for co-occurring disorders clinical positions; makes recommendations concerning how interviews can be conducted to maximize information about applicants' knowledge and experience concerning co-occurring disorders treatment; and discusses how the decision-making process can be most effective.

Most agencies have standardized application forms that fulfill all the essential and mandated data elements that must be collected regarding future employees. This type of information ranges from name and address to the applicant's specialized licenses or certifications. Program managers who hire individuals to provide co-occurring disorders clinical services must ensure that their application form includes the following four important pieces of background information: (1) experience providing co-occurring treatment services; (2) type of co-occurring treatment population worked with and the work setting; (3) specific treatment functions performed with the clients; and (4) specific education and training the applicant has had concerning co-occurring treatment. These questions can be woven either into other similar questions on the application form or attached as a supplement to it.

Applicants can realistically accomplish the following during an interview:

- highlight their co-occurring disorders education, training, and treatment backgrounds;
- demonstrate their knowledge about the treatment of such disorders;
- show their ability to diagnose and develop treatment plans for this population; and
- present a limited picture of how they interact with others.

Depending on the size of the program and the size of the applicant pool, interviews may be structured as an interaction between the applicant and a single interviewer; an interaction between the applicant and an interview panel; or an interaction between several applicants and an individual or interview panel (group interview). Group interviews are usually used to reduce the applicant pool to a more manageable size. Interviews are usually conducted face to face, but many are now being conducted by phone or via the Internet.

In order for interviews to obtain the clearest picture of candidates, the questions must be specific enough to ensure that vague answers will not suffice. Appendix B provides sample interview questions that can be used to allow applicants to expand on the information they provided on the application form concerning their education, training, and experience with co-occurring disorders. Appendix B also provides sample interview questions that address the applicant's knowledge of the nature of co-occurring disorders and the best treatment practices for this population, as well as providing a client scenario and sample questions that allow applicants to demonstrate their ability to make initial diagnostic assessments and treatment plans. Because these questions take some time to think about, they should be either given to the applicant ahead of time or be answered as a written exercise following the formal portion of the interview. Including such questions in the interview will provide the broadest picture possible of the applicants.

Once all the interviews are completed, a decision must be made concerning which applicants should be hired. I have found six applicant characteristics useful in making this decision. These characteristics are experience, knowledge, ability and willingness to learn the job, and general temperament and apparent stability. Information concerning these characteristics comes from the application form, responses to the interview questions, personal interactions during the interviews, and from reference checks. Appendix B provides a sample work sheet that can be used to evaluate each applicant on these four dimensions and provide comparisons among individuals.

Experience involves hands-on clinical work with individuals with co-occurring disorders. The longer the experience the higher the applicant would score on the scale. Also contributing to a higher score on this scale is experience in providing these services to the specific subgroup that the program treats, experience in the treatment modality that the program uses, and in the same treatment setting that the program operates. A program providing co-occurring disorders treatment services for Subgroup IV (high psychiatric symptoms and high substance use symptoms) would give an applicant who has experience working with Subgroup III (high substance abuse symptoms, low psychiatric symptoms) in a residential setting a lower score than an applicant who had worked with this population in an outpatient setting.

Knowledge involves the ability to answer the interview questions concerning diagnostic and treatment techniques in a thorough and comprehensive manner. An applicant who is able to articulate how co-occurring disorders treatment is the same as and different from traditional substance abuse treatment and describes how this plays out in working with clients will score higher on this dimension than an applicant who knows the buzzwords about treating this population but has difficulty articulating how these changes may apply in day-to-day treatment interventions.

Ability to learn the job involves demonstrating psychological intelligence and sophistication, intuitiveness about working with this population, and enthusiasm and interest in working with the population. An applicant who has no experience working with this population but expresses a definite interest in doing so, demonstrates a strong knowledge of how therapy works, and intuitively makes treatment suggestions that would be appropriate for this population would score higher on this dimension than an applicant who expresses a similar interest to work with this population but shows little insight into their treatment needs.

General temperament and apparent stability can be assessed from observations made during the interview. Did the applicant arrive on time for the interview? Is there a history of many job changes? Do the person's responses to interview questions demonstrate treatment flexibility, creativity, and optimism and respectfulness toward clients? Do references describe a cooperative individual? Does the applicant appear psychologically stable? An applicant who arrives on time, has a stable work history, and demonstrates an apparent temperament of optimism and creativity would score higher on this dimension than an applicant who is ten minutes late for the interview and whose current employer indicates that there had been some conflict between this individual and another staff member.

Using a scale of one to ten for each of these dimensions is arbitrary, but the scaling can serve as helpful benchmarks for hiring decisions. In theory each dimension is equal in importance, yet some may be more important in certain situations than others. For example, one applicant has some experience working with individuals with co-occurring disorders, has had significant training in the treatment of this population, and expresses enthusiasm for working with the population. Another applicant has no experience working with this population, no training in their treatment, but does express a strong interest in learning to work with these individuals. In regard to these three dimensions, the first applicant will score much higher on two of the three categories. However, the first applicant presents in a manner that makes the interviewers question her ability to work effectively as a team member and the reference check results in vague responses concerning this issue. The second applicant clearly demonstrates strong therapy skills and a very pleasant and cooperative personality. In this instance the program manager decides to hire the second applicant, even though she is less experienced and has less training, because the manager belives she will be able to learn the job and will be a better fit for the team approach used by the program. The applicant assessment form provides valuable information for hiring decisions but the scales should never be used as the sole criterion for these decisions.

DEVELOPING AND IMPLEMENTING TRAINING PROGRAMS

When beginning to provide co-occurring disorders treatment services, most staff members will not have all the knowledge, skills, and attitudes necessary to be effective with this population. Program management must therefore develop and implement training programs for their staff that cover basic values and philosophies, essential knowledge, and specific assessment and treatment skills necessary to treat this population. Implementing such staff training programs involves the following four steps:

1. Identifying staff training needs
2. Deciding on training structure
3. Determining who will provide the training
4. Evaluating training effectiveness

Identifying Staff Training Needs

Staff members working with co-occurring disorders bring different levels of experience, knowledge, and skills to the job. Before a training program is implemented the exact training needs of the staff must be ascertained. Appendix C is a sample training needs assessment that can be used or modified to identify staff training needs. This self-assessment tool measures perceived levels of knowledge and abilities and the specific interest in acquiring this information and these skills. In general, staff members who self-report knowledge and skill levels below IV for any topic should be targeted for training in those areas. If motivation for training in any area is low, then training will need to include a motivation component that justifies the need for this training. The form also provides the opportunity for the clinical supervisor to have input into this needs assessment process if desired. The needs assessment can be used to assess the training needs of all program staff or the training needs of newly hired staff members. Once training needs are identified, a decision must be made concerning the structure of the training.

Deciding on Training Structure

Training programs can be designed for presentation in group settings or for a single individual. Obviously, training for just one individual will be designed to specifically meet that person's needs. Alhough it is important to individualize instruction as much as possible, budgetary and time restrictions usually require use of group format. The key to making the group format as individualized as possible is to use the needs assessment process previously discussed to determine which staff members would benefit most from particular instruction. For example, two staff members report that they have sufficient skill levels in conducting assessments and developing treatment plans for individuals with co-occurring disorders, while seven report they do not have skills in this area. The clinical supervisor agrees with this assessment, so only the seven reporting inadequate skills would be targeted for the training. In another example, a one-day training is offered on providing individual, group, and family treatment interventions for individuals with co-occurring disorders. Staff members report differing degrees of expertise in each of these treatment modalities, but none report expertise in all, so it is decided to send all staff to the training because each will benefit from some portion of it. The individual training format is normally used when there are not enough staff members who need a particular skill to form a group. Often this format uses individual supervision, professional readings, or another staff member to achieve the needed training. Examples of this are the use of individual clinical supervision to improve a staff member's ability to make diagnostic assessments of co-occurring disorders, or arranging for a staff member to meet regularly with another therapist to discuss how to be an effective case manager for this population. Once the training structure has been determined, which is often a mix of group and individual training formats, it must be decided who will provide the training.

Determining Who Will Provide the Training

Training can be accomplished by agency staff, hired consultants, conference attendance, or outside programs. The method used is normally based on internal staff expertise and the amount of training money available. Most programs will use some mixture of these resources. When few staff members have a particular training need the supervisory process usually provides the needed training; when many staff members have a particular training need, an outside trainer or consultant is often brought in or staff are sent to conferences or specialized training programs. For example, a new staff member is hired who has not worked with this population before and thus does not know the basics of treating the agency's population. Since other staff do not have this training need, the new staff member is paired up with an experienced clinician to observe how intakes are conducted, how groups are led, and how case management activities are carried out. The experienced therapist is readily available to answer any questions and can provide immediate feedback. This process is further reinforced by biweekly clinical supervision and continues until the new staff member has the basic skills to work with the program's population.

In another instance, management has decided to add a family treatment component to its program. The staff has little experience or training in providing this modality, so a family treatment consultant is hired. The consultant first provides basic training for all the staff about family interventions, and then meets with them weekly for a year to reinforce the training and provide clinical supervision concerning family interventions.

Evaluating Training Effectiveness

Since program managers may commit a great deal of staff time and money to these training procedures, they will need to know how effective they are. Many methods can be used for measuring program effectiveness. The most common measures include increase in knowledge; self-reports of increased feelings of competency; clinical supervisor's observations of increased skills; or improved client outcomes.

Knowledge increase measures usually involve pre- and post-tests that determine what information participants obtained from the training. Measures of increased beliefs in competency are usually self-reports that training participants complete at the end of training and periodically thereafter. Clinical supervision measures are completed by the clinical supervisors and compare the effectiveness of a clinician at performing a task prior to the training and at sometime thereafter (often six months). Improved client outcome measures are normally tied to a program's performance and outcome measures (see Chapter 10 for commonly used measures) and usually compare changes in these measures annually. Program managers can use one or more of these measures to gauge the effectiveness of their training programs.

It is important that programs that provide co-occurring treatment services develop orientation training for all new staff that covers the basics of treating this population, provides regular internal ongoing training on co-occurring disorders topics, and sets aside enough funds to allow staff members to attend at least one outside training per year. Also, identifying and providing for the training needs of staff is an ongoing process. Therefore, I recommend that any program providing co-occurring treatment services establish a training committee composed of clinical and supervisory staff who at least annually assess the training needs of staff, provide ongoing internal training, and advocate for funds to attend outside training.

CONCLUSION

This chapter focused on the hiring and development of clinical service providers of programs offering treatment services for individuals with co-occurring disorders. The chapter reviewed the essential knowledge, skills, and characteristics that staff must have to provide effective treatment services to this population. Recommendations were made concerning the selection process for new staff and methods outlined for developing and implementing a staff training program. The next chapter focuses on the issues involved in providing effective clinical supervision for these direct service providers.

Chapter 7

Clinical Supervision of Treatment Services for Co-Occurring Disorders

Although a great deal of professional literature focuses on the supervision of staff treating either mental health or substance use disorders (Bernard and Goodyear, 1992; Borders and Leddick, 1987; Machell, 1987; McDaniel, Weber, and McKeever, 1983; Powell and Brodsky, 2004; Worthington, 1987), few focus on supervising staff who treat clients with co-occurring disorders (Hendrickson, Schmal, and Ekleberry, 2004; Hendrickson et al., 1999). Effective clinical supervision plays a critical role in ensuring that effective and appropriate treatment services are provided to this population and also plays a critical role in staff development. This chapter reviews the qualities of an effective clinical supervisor of co-occurring disorders treatment services, discusses options for establishing a supervisory structure for these services, presents twelve common supervisory issues and makes recommendations for addressing them, and describes ways to develop a supervision process.

QUALITIES OF AN EFFECTIVE CLINICAL SUPERVISOR

The effective clinical supervisor for staff providing treatment services for individuals with co-occurring disorders must possess the following seven important supervisory qualities:

- willingness to exercise leadership;
- advocating for the program's clinical services;
- being readily available to clinical staff;
- assisting staff in remaining calm and focused in their clinical work;

- providing supervisory interventions that are flexible, creative, or directive depending on the need at the time;
- having knowledge of best practices for this population; and
- having experience providing treatment services to these individuals with co-occurring disorders.

The following describes each of these qualities in detail.

Willingness to Exercise Leadership

Leadership is a term often used, despite little consensus regarding its definition. Different leadership traits are needed for different types of leadership roles. Traits that make a combat leader effective might not be traits that make an effective chairperson of a consensus panel. The two leadership traits that clinical supervisors for co-occurring disorders treatment services must possess are (1) the ability to inspire and (2) the willingness to speak honestly to the clinical staff about the clients they work with, the services they provide, and management decisions with which they must live. To inspire means helping staff believe they are capable of effecting change; speaking honestly means placing trust in the staff's ability to comprehend the big picture of their program and its treatment environment. The following are examples of these qualities.

Ability to Inspire

If staff are to work effectively with clients who have multiple problems and a history of multiple treatment failures, they must believe in themselves as clinicians. A supervisor of these services must emphasize clinical successes and frame clinical failures as learning opportunities. For example, a client who has never participated in treatment for more than three weeks stays in treatment for five months before relapsing and leaving treatment. In this instance the supervisor points out to the staff members who worked with this client that no other clinical staff had been able to promote this level of treatment engagement before. The supervisor would also want to know from these clinicians which skills and abilities they possess that promoted such a lengthy engagement. The treatment event is then rightly framed in the minds of the staff as a success instead of a failure.

In another instance, a client relapses, becomes psychotic, and is hospitalized. During the clinical review of the case it becomes apparent that several warning signs had not been adequately addressed by the client's therapist. The client had reported an increasing frequency of drug-using dreams, missed some scheduled appointments, and a third-party report indicated that the client was not taking medication as prescribed. However, the clinician, who was fairly new to the program, did not explore ways of addressing these issues or intensifying treatment during normal supervision. The supervisor, instead of focusing on what the staff member did incorrectly (which was already clearly apparent to that clinician), explored how the case might have been handled differently so that relapse and hospitalization could have been prevented. Focusing on what could have been done differently creates a learning environment and increases the clinician's confidence to handle a similar situation in the future.

Speaking Honestly

Speaking directly and honestly to clinical staff concerning clients, services, and management implies that the clinical supervisor must trust them to be professional, have a mature view of the world, and behave in that mature manner. For example, new forms are continuously added to most treatment programs' documentation systems. Often these forms collect duplicate information, exist only because the data is required by some licensing or funding source, and seldom are seen as being useful to the staff's clinical work. When new forms are introduced, there is normally an uproar among the staff and they have a need to restate the above realities. Supervisors who are honest and direct will allow this uproar for a short while so that staff members can vent frustration. These supervisors will also in no way attempt to honey coat or put a positive spin on the form unless they honestly believe it, and will acknowledge that much of what the staff is saying is true. However, at some point in this process the supervisor must simply say it is unfortunate that they have to do it, but the form must be completed to meet licensure requirements. Handling the situation in such a manner allows the staff and the supervisor to be honest about their feelings, but at the same time creates the expectation that all are capable of understanding the complexities of working in systems and acting in a mature manner.

In another instance, a percentage of an outpatient co-occurring disorders treatment program's clients are in need of residential treatment; however, no such services are available to them. Honest supervisors will quickly acknowledge to staff that some clients are not receiving the level of treatment they need. The supervisor will also honestly share the likelihood of why or why not such services may be established. In this case the supervisor will also share that management had decided it was better to provide some services to these clients rather than none. Occasionally a staff member will not behave in a mature or professional manner and the supervisor gets burned by the honesty; in general, the empowerment that staff members experience when let into the entire process will greatly outweigh the inappropriate behavior of a few. The supervisor must have the ego to handle these occasional burns. To possess these two traits, supervisors must truly see the world in a positive and competency-based way and be willing to communicate to staff that they trust them to carry out their clinical functions even when they do not want to.

Advocating for the Program's Clinical Services

Clinical supervisors must always balance two loyalties that at times conflict. They have loyalty to the program, being part of the management team, and loyalty to the clinical services they supervise. More often than not, the program and clinical needs are congruent, but at times they come into conflict. For example, to meet state standards, a program must update its policy and procedures manual. This is normally the responsibility of the management team, but two management positions are currently vacant and several other critical documents with immediate deadlines must be completed. In response to this situation, the program manager decides that a staff work group will be established to update the policy and procedures manual. All but one of the staff members selected for this work group are clinicians and it appears that this work group's task will be a fairly time-consuming one. Obviously, in order to complete the policies and procedures manual some level of clinical services will need to be curtailed.

In such situations, the clinical supervisor must act as the advocate for the program's clinical services. If no advocate is available at the management level for clinical services then they begin to take a backseat to the administrative requirements of the program. Ultimately this will lead to a reduction in the quality of clinical services and eventually may place the program's survival at risk. In this situation the clinical supervisor acknowledges that the manual must be completed but rightly points out that the heavy investment of clinical staff time on the work group will reduce clinical services. The supervisor questions the wisdom of this and wonders if other remedies have been explored, such as obtaining an extension of the manual's due date because of vacant management positions, or hiring a consultant with the unspent vacant positions money to create the manual. Although it might seem as if the clinical supervisor is not being a team player, in fact the supervisor is fulfilling the primary function of this position by informing the rest of the management team how their decisions impact clinical services. When conflict exists between clinical services and other aspects of a treatment program, the clinical supervisor is most loyal to the program when lobbying for minimum impact on clinical services.

Ready Availability to Clinical Staff

Many clinical questions arise when staff is dealing with clients who have multiple problems. The staff must feel that they have ready access to clinical supervision and support when these questions arise in order not to experience undue anxiety. Thus clinical supervisors of services for individuals with co-occurring disorders must be easily available to their staff. A supervisor with this quality establishes both formal and informal channels of supervision. For example, the supervisor establishes a formal structure for all staff that involves at least a once-a-week supervision. This structure could be individual, group, or a mixture of both depending on needs of the staff. The supervisor will also ensure that staff members believe that they can come at any time and discuss anything about a case, that the decision to seek supervision is based on need, and not because they are bothering the supervisor. The supervisor will say such things as, "You can come and talk about a case anytime," or "the only dumb question is the one not asked." Such supervisors will also ensure that every day some time is available for staff supervision by either themselves or a backup supervisor. The meta-message being communicated by all these actions is that supervision is an important and valuable part of these services. In many ways this supervisory quality is an extension of the previous one involving advocating for clinical services.

Creating a Calm and Focused Treatment Environment

Individuals with co-occurring disorders often bring multiple, complicated, and interacting problems to the treatment environment. When staff encounter clients with such multiple treatment needs they often feel overwhelmed and become anxious and unclear concerning treatment direction. It is important that the clinical supervisor be able to assist staff in maintaining an overall clinical picture of the client and not get caught up in the day-to-day changes that the client may experience. Also it is important that the supervisor helps staff develop clear and focused treatment plans for the multiple problems they encounter. For example, a staff member who has a client who periodically relapses and becomes suicidal might get very anxious when this occurs. Supervisors who are calm and focused will help the staff frame such events as a time-limited crisis that can be successfully resolved with prearranged intervention strategies. The supervisor points out that this is the client's pattern, that the crisis has been successfully dealt with several times, the treatment plan has specific interventions to be used when this occurs, and the clinician is not alone with this client; others are available to help too. By pointing out these realities to the clinician, the supervisor helps create a calmer treatment environment by incorporating the entire treatment system into the therapist's support system. Also, by pointing out that a focused and effective treatment plan is in place, this becomes the road map to follow to reduce anxiety. Obviously, in instances where a clear treatment is not in place for a specific treatment issue, then supervisors with this quality will help clinical staff develop one and guide them through its implementation. Several common supervisory issues discussed later in this chapter deal more specifically with staff anxiety management and treatment plan development.

Individualized Supervisory Interventions

Staff providing treatment services for individuals with co-occurring disorders will have a wide range of experience providing treatment to this population, and their clients will have a wide range of treatment needs. Thus every staff member will need a somewhat different type of supervision, and each client will need a slightly different type of treatment. To handle these differences, clinical supervisors of this treatment population must use a mixture of flexibility, creativity, and direction to individualize supervisory interventions. For example, a supervisor with this quality may choose to be very directive with an inexperienced therapist concerning types of interventions to use, but be collegial concerning choice of interventions with a seasoned therapist. In another instance, the supervisor might suggest that a client with antisocial personality traits not be allowed to miss any treatment sessions, while suggesting for another client with paranoid symptoms that there should be flexibility concerning treatment attendance. In still another example, the supervisor helps a staff member create an outpatient alcohol detoxification strategy for a client who will not be accepted by the local detoxification program because of his prescribed use of an addicting anti-anxiety medication for his severe anxiety symptoms. Supervisors providing clinical supervision for this population must have the capacity to individualize their supervisory strategies to effectively support staff with a wide range of professional experience working with clients who have multiple problems.

Knowledge of Best Treatment Practices

Because this population lacks experienced clinical supervisors, it is possible that a supervisor could be hired into such a position without ever having worked with or supervised staff working with co-occurring disorders. In those instances, these supervisors will bring knowledge concerning best practices for substance abuse or mental health treatment, but not necessarily both. The quality needed by supervisors in such instances is the willingness to learn the best practices for this population and the willingness to put aside old beliefs when they run counter to these best practices. For example, right after a new supervisor who is inexperienced in working with co-occurring disorders is hired, she reads as much literature about this population as possible, arranges to attend several conferences on treating these individuals, and visits several programs providing such services to get advice from their clinical supervisors.

In another example, an individual who has worked in the substance abuse field for more than twenty years is hired as a supervisor for a new co-occurring disorders treatment program that provides services for individuals with severe substance use and psychiatric symptoms. His prior experience had taught him to wait before providing medication for clients using or withdrawing from alcohol and other drugs. However, he is willing to change this belief based on feedback from other program staff who are more experienced with this population as well as from his own observations of these clients. It is not always possible to hire a supervisor who knows all the best practices for treating this population, but it will be necessary to hire a supervisor who is willing to learn them and be able to change long-held beliefs.

Experience Providing Clinical Services to This Population

As in the case of best practices, a program may not be able to find a capable supervisor who is experienced in treating individuals with co-occurring disorders. However, a clinical supervisor must know what it is like to sit in the therapy room with these clients, what their process of change is like, and what is likely to happen in certain situations. Without this knowledge, supervisors cannot demonstrate that they have an understanding of their staff's real world. If the staff believes that the supervisor is ignorant of their working world, then all supervisory feedback is viewed skeptically. This skepticism can undermine the supervisory process even when it is appropriate, accurate, and therapeutically helpful. Thus supervisors without experience working with this population must obtain this experience to be effective. For example, a supervisor is hired by a program that works with individuals who have high substance abuse symptoms and low mental health symptoms. This supervisor brings supervisory experience in a program for treating the seriously mentally ill and direct service experience in a substance abuse prevention program, but has never worked with individuals with co-occurring high substance use and low psychiatric symptoms. The quality looked for in this supervisor is the willingness to obtain the necessary experience. In this instance, the new supervisor decides to both co-lead a treatment group and carry a small caseload of these clients for at least a year to gain the necessary experience. It is not always possible to hire a supervisor who has experience treating this population, but it will be necessary to hire a supervisor who is willing to obtain this experience.

ESTABLISHING A SUPERVISORY STRUCTURE

When establishing a clinical supervision structure several questions must be answered. These questions are (1) how often will supervision be held? (2) what format will it use? (3) how many persons will participate in it? and (4) what will its focus be? Several program and individual factors often dictate how these questions are answered. These factors include the following:

- the size of the organization;
- the number of employees supervised;
- the number and type of clients served;
- other roles and functions the clinical supervisor must perform;
- the staff's supervisory needs; and
- the supervisor's supervisory philosophy.

Because of these differences, a variety of clinical supervisory structures will be found in programs providing co-occurring disorders treatment services. One supervisory structure may emphasize individual supervision while another may primarily use group supervision; one supervisory structure might thoroughly review every case once a week while another will meet every two weeks and only review cases that staff feel they are having trouble with. In still another supervisory structure, only clinical issues are addressed while in another both clinical and administrative issues are addressed at the meetings. Not one supervisory structure fits all co-occurring treatment programs; however, there is one that will best fit the supervisory needs of a particular program. The purpose of this section is to discuss the issues involved in selecting a supervisory structure.

Supervisory structures will differ, but the goal of the structure is always the same: it ensures that the clients' treatment needs are met and that they are within the supervisory capabilities of the program. The treatment needs of clients are met when they receive state-of-the-art interventions and their therapist is genuinely able to communicate to them that they have the ability to change. To provide state-of-the-art and competency-focused treatment, supervision must help clinicians examine their treatment interventions to see if they are following accepted practices for this population and provide the opportunity for them to express, explore, and resolve their frustrations about clients who are not doing well. To accomplish this, the supervisory structure must include formal and informal supervision and ongoing training. Formal supervision is a prescribed time when clinical issues will be discussed and examined; informal supervision is the process of a therapist coming to a supervisor outside this prescribed time to discuss a clinical issue. For example, the intervention strategy agreed to for a case during formal supervision becomes inappropriate because of new third-party information. Instead of waiting for the next scheduled supervisory session, the therapist seeks out the supervisor in order to modify the intervention strategy. While supervision focuses on specific intervention strategies, ongoing training provides the clinical staff with necessary knowledge and skills to upgrade their clinical practices to state-of-the-art treatment. Issues that commonly need formal and informal supervision in co-occurring disorders treatment programs are discussed in the next section of this chapter.

The supervisory capacity of a program is the amount of time that can be dedicated solely to clinical supervision and is generally dictated by the program size. Smaller programs usually have less time to dedicate to supervisory activities because the staffs in these smaller programs often perform multiple functions. It would not be uncommon for a manager of a smaller program to also be the clinical supervisor. This individual must perform both management and supervisory functions. In such a case the supervisory structure could probably be more group oriented than individual; formal supervision might occur less than once a week with informal and peer supervision playing a bigger part in the supervisory process; and administrative supervision would probably occur conjointly with clinical supervision. Ongoing training would also probably be an outside-the-agency activity, or outside consultants would be brought in to perform this function. On the other hand, a larger treatment program might have a staff member whose sole function is to provide clinical supervision. In this instance the supervisory structure would probably include formalized individual and group supervision activities and informal supervision would probably also be available. Peer supervision would play a much smaller part in this supervisory process. In addition, the clinical supervisor might be responsible for developing in-house clinical training programs and for actually providing many of these trainings. Although all supervisory structures must ensure that staff receive adequate formal and informal supervision and ongoing training, the way it is shaped and formed will vary greatly among programs, with program size often being the key factor.

COMMON SUPERVISORY ISSUES

Twelve common supervisory issues arise periodically when clinical services are being offered to individuals with co-occurring disorders. These issues involve client needs, staff needs, and program/system needs. Some are similar to normal substance abuse and mental health supervisory concerns and some are unique to services for co-occurring disorders. All must be adequately dealt with if treatment services are to be effective and comprehensive. The following is a description of each supervisory issue and recommendations concerning how each can be best addressed.

Dealing with Diverse Treatment Needs

Therapists working with clients with co-occurring disorders will encounter a wide range of mental health and substance abuse treatment issues. Substance use disorders may range from alcohol abuse to narcotics dependence and mental health disorders might range from generalized anxiety disorder to schizophrenia. Because this population presents with such a wide variety of symptoms, treatment intervention strategies must be tailored to the individual needs of each client. Some clients can easily achieve abstinence and tolerate intensive confrontational therapy, while other clients lack the necessary skills to initially achieve abstinence and decompensate quickly if confrontation is too intense.

The role of supervision when encountering this issue is twofold. The first is to teach clinicians to develop individualized treatment plans that take into consideration the differences that their clients have in symptom level, level of impairment, and coping skills. When the treatment plan accurately mirrors the treatment needs and capacities of the client, the chances of a successful treatment outcome are significantly increased. The second is to familiarize staff with subgroup models for this population as discussed in Chapters 2 and 3. By organizing this population into more heterogeneous clusters with similar treatment needs, the time needed to develop individualized treatment plans can be reduced.

Defining Treatment Goals

For treatment interventions to have a coherent direction, they must have clear and concise goals. The multitude of problems that this population presents is often overwhelming and can create confusion concerning which issues to treat and when to treat them. For example, a client might present with a recent suicide attempt, delusions and hallucinations, sexual identity confusion, anger, mistrust, possible HIV and hepatitis C, alcohol dependence, and cannabis, cocaine, and narcotic abuse. This can be a very intimidating picture even for an experienced treatment professional. When a clinician is unclear about the direction and focus of treatment, little chance exists for success.

The role of supervision in this instance is to help clinicians develop clear and concise treatment goals for their treatment interventions. Table 7.1 presents treatment goals recommended by Hendrickson, Schmal, and Ekleberry (2004) for caseloads that include individuals with co-occurring disorders. These treatment goals are based on the type of disorders that clients have. Using this model can provide therapists with guidance when they encounter a client with multiple disorders and treatment needs, because ultimately the treatment goals will be abstinence, psychiatric stability, and/or interpersonal stability. Although many treatment objectives must be met before these goals can be achieved, having clear and concise long-term goals helps therapists identify the specific objectives and treatment interventions that need to be included in their treatment plan.

TABLE 7.1. Treatment Goals

Disorder Type	Treatment Goals
MH Disorders Only	Psychiatric Stability
SA Disorders Only	Abstinence (Dependency Disorders) Nonproblematic Substance Use (Abuse Disorders)
SA and MH Disorders	Abstinence and Psychiatric Stability
SA and Personality Disorders	Abstinence and Interpersonal Stability
SA, MH, and Personality Disorders	Abstinence, Psychiatric Stability, and Interpersonal Stability

Identifying the Views of Family/Peer Networks Concerning Treatment

Families and peers have significant influence on the behavior of clients. They can promote, support, hinder, or undermine new behaviors. A therapist, however, cannot determine the full extent of this impact without actually interacting with these individuals. For example, a client with major depressive disorder and alcohol and cocaine dependence who had been abstinent and psychiatrically stable for four months suddenly begins missing a few scheduled appointments and not going as frequently to her self-help groups. She tells her therapist only that she is experiencing some family problems. The therapist is unclear as to whether she is using this as an excuse, or if there are real problems, and if so, what they are, and how they might impact her recovery.

The role of supervision in this instance is to help the staff member identify how to involve the family in the treatment process. Numerous intervention processes have been proposed for involving the family in mental health, substance abuse, or co-occurring disorders treatment (Hendrickson, Schmal, and Ekleberry, 2004; McCollum and Trotter, 2001), so it is important that the supervisor is familiar with these and is willing to share this information with the staff member working with this client. In this instance, the supervisor works first to help the therapist understand how important it is to get detailed information about these stated family problems and then help the therapist strategize how to obtain this information. After some resistance, the client finally shares with the therapist that her family thinks she is spending too much of her time in treatment activities and is against her taking antidepressant medication. The client also shares that she had received some feedback at her self-help groups that taking medication for a long time might interfere with her recovery. Once the issue of family problems has been clarified, the supervisor can work with the therapist on how to involve the family more positively in the treatment process and how to help the client deal with conflicting treatment recommendations.

Identifying Staff Training Needs

Usually clinicians who work with clients with multiple diagnoses have expertise in treating either substance use or mental health disorders, but not both. To ensure that these clients receive effective treatment, supervisors need to identify their clinical staff's knowledge and skills gaps and promote training opportunities to fill these gaps. Table 6.1 in Chapter 6 presents the knowledge and skills that clinicians working with this population most often need to add to their professional repertoire. Supervisors can also use the proposed training assessment tool presented in Chapter 6 to identify the training needs of their staff.

Once supervisors identify these needs, they can lobby for or designate agency training money to send staff to specialized trainings or hire experts to conduct training within the agency. This method allows numerous staff members to attend the sessions concurrently and process their understanding of the new information with one another. This strategy also is especially cost-effective and places limited demands on staff time. On the other hand, one-time training sessions tend to increase knowledge more than skills and offer no reinforcement of newly acquired information; as a result, staff members often return to old practices.

A second method of increasing staff competencies is to have clinical staff with different expertise co-lead a group. Together, both clinicians can effectively address all the substance abuse and mental health issues that arise in the group and through observations of how the other therapist handles certain situations and from the feedback they give each other, both begin to develop the expertise needed to treat multiple disorders. The strength of this method is that multineed clients have their treatment needs met while the clinicians are still developing the necessary competencies to effectively treat them. It also allows staff to be both experts and students at the same time. On the other hand, this method requires two staff members to work collaboratively and to have the interest and motivation to learn new competencies. Such groups also often require staff to have more than one supervisor, so a multiple supervisory arrangement needs to be worked out (see the supervision issue of system blending, p. 143). Simply having individuals with different expertise on a multidisciplinary team seldom increases the competencies of other team staff unless the other staff members are required to work with clients with multiple disorders and have the opportunity to observe integrated treatment skills in action.

The third method is to integrate mental health and substance abuse issues into all aspects of the supervisory process and to address all the mental health and substance use concerns regarding assessment, treatment plans, and intervention strategies in clinical discussions. This of course requires the supervisor to have expertise in both of these areas. When this is not the case, an expert can be consulted to both upgrade the supervisor's expertise and provide clinical guidance for the staff. Although any of these methods would be helpful in increasing staff competencies, if they all were used concurrently, staff would quickly acquire new attitudes, knowledge, and skills.

Helping Staff Manage Function and Role Shifts

The multiple treatment and support needs of clients with co-occurring disorders often require clinicians to perform a wide variety of functions and roles. For example, a therapist with a client with alcohol dependence and schizoaffective disorders at times provides individual, group, or family therapy for this client; at other times she performs case management or advocacy functions. These shifts in roles and functions are often confusing for clinicians and may run counter to some of their professional training. It is not uncommon to hear a clinician ask, "Am I a therapist, a case manager, or a community advocate?"

When clinicians are struggling with this issue, supervisors need to help them answer "yes, yes, yes" to these questions. Supervisors can help by connecting specific clinical tasks to treatment goals. The supervisor will need to point out that to promote the goals of abstinence, psychiatric stability, and/or interpersonal stability, the clinician as a group therapist must promote acceptance of the disorders and a desire for abstinence plus medication compliance. However, the therapist also must be a case manager when helping the client complete all the necessary forms to ensure medication availability, and a community advocate when promoting a client's acceptance into a supportive housing program. Should any of these tasks not be performed, the chance of treatment success is reduced. In addition, one role or function is not more important than another in determining the ultimate success of treatment.

Maintaining a Positive View Concerning the Potential for Change

Many clients with serious impairments have had a number of previous treatments and other failures in life. Therapists encountering such clients may become pessimistic about their ability to provide successful treatment. In this case, supervisors need to focus on the problems and failures that reinforce this pessimistic point of view for both the therapist and the client. For example, a client enters treatment with a history of discontinuing medication that controls the symptoms of his bipolar disorder, then returns to alcohol use to reduce some of the emerging manic symptoms, and ends up being hospitalized. Soon after beginning treatment, the client reports that he does not think his medication is helping. The therapist immediately assumes that the client has begun his same old pattern over again and tells his supervisor that he is not going to put much effort into the case because the client is on the way to the hospital again.

In such situations, the supervisor needs to promote competency-based interventions, which are described in Chapter 2. These interventions focus on clients' strengths and positive experiences with therapy, and promote a sense of optimism that even more change is possible. In this case, the supervisor points out that the client is currently coming to therapy and taking his medication and asks the clinician what skills or motivation the client might have that allowed him to be medication compliant and abstinent for periods of time. How could these be used to either interrupt the relapse cycle or at least extend the period of stability? By asking such questions the view that change is possible greatly increases. Therapists often initially resist competency-based supervisory strategies because they feel too "Pollyanna-ish" or they may see the supervisor as naive, so supervisors often have to persist in using this type of intervention. Supervisors can also help clinicians develop competency-based skills by having them incorporate client strengths into all treatment plans, especially for individuals about whom they are pessimistic. Supervisors can monitor the level of pessimism by asking clinicians to always include the client's prognosis in their clinical discussions. To ensure that the treatment plans reflect realistic and achievable goals for the client in the previous case, the supervisor may suggest that the initial goals be an increase in how long the client is medication compliant and abstinent and a decrease in the time spent in relapse and in the hospital. In doing so, success is defined as any positive change, and change can promote more change.

Ensuring Integrated Treatment

Providing effective integrated treatment involves being aware of and addressing how multiple disorders interact with one another and how their interactions affect a client. Chapter 2 offers a detailed description of integrated treatment. For example, during a clinical supervision session with a therapist who has a client with social phobia and cannabis abuse disorders and occasional panic attacks, the therapist discusses how she has been working with the anxiety disorders, both with medication and behavior intervention. However, the client perceives little change in symptoms. The therapist does not discuss how she is addressing the marijuana use at all, therefore the supervisor needs to introduce that issue into supervision.

To help clinicians become proficient in providing integrated treatment, supervisors must ensure that treatment plans for clients with multiple disorders include problem statements and treatment goals and objectives for each disorder. In supervision, the supervisor can ask therapists to discuss how their treatment interventions address the treatment goals for each disorder. A third strategy is to occasionally ask the therapist what she thinks will happen to one disorder if the symptoms of the other disorder increase or decrease. In this example, the supervisor needs to ask about the status of the client's marijuana use, the treatment goals for that disorder, the intervention strategies the therapist is using to accomplish these goals, and how the marijuana use might affect the lack of decrease in psychiatric symptoms. Such questions help bring into focus actions to address all the disorders and how these disorders might affect one another.

Dealing with Anxiety and Unhelpful Clinical Behavior

Many clients with multiple disorders are unable or unwilling initially to work toward the treatment goals of abstinence or psychiatric or interpersonal stability. Sometimes the level of client symptoms and/or impairments can lead to life-threatening situations. In fact, many clients with multiple disorders die prematurely, either by their own hands or because of the consequences of their behavior. Blumenthal (1988) reports that 90 percent of adults who commit suicide have a mental disorder and up to 80 percent have a substance use disorder. Working with such clients can create a great deal of anxiety for therapists and cause either over-functioning or expressions of hostility toward a client. For example, a client has schizoaffective, alcohol dependence, and opioid abuse disorders, and is also positive for HIV and hepatitis C. This client is only partially compliant with his medications for both his mental health and medical disorders. He also has a history of becoming paranoid and getting into fights in which he has been seriously injured. At this point, the therapist has no leverage to use to promote abstinence or medication compliance. The only action the client is willing to perform regularly is to see the therapist individually on a weekly basis.

Supervisors can help clinicians deal more effectively with anxiety and inappropriate behavior by promoting clear and appropriate therapeutic boundaries and by helping them design interventions that match best treatment practices with client readiness. In the previous example, the therapist comes to supervision very anxious about this client. He rightly believes that the client's life is in jeopardy, if not immediately, certainly in the long run. He is also angry and frustrated with the client concerning treatment noncompliance. The therapist really wants a magic intervention strategy from supervision that will enlighten and motivate the client to become treatment compliant. The supervisor must first acknowledge the reality that the therapist is dealing with a client who might die, but the responsibility for that does not lie with the therapist alone. The supervisor, other professionals involved in the client's treatment, and the client also have responsibilities concerning the outcome of treatment. By doing this, the burden of the case is lightened for the therapist.

The supervisor's next step is to point out that the client has found something helpful in seeing the therapist because he attends treatment once a week. Since no outside leverage is available, the supervisor then helps the therapist identify short-term achievable goals that can form the basis for eventually achieving the long-term goals. Examples of these goals include getting the client to attend a psychoeducation group about either his mental health or medical disorders or encouraging the client to take his medication more frequently. Such strategies begin to help the therapist see that something positive is already happening in therapy and that change is possible. The supervisor should also point out that the client has only marginally engaged with treatment and that other therapists would not be achieving any different results at this stage of recovery. Finally, the supervisor can help the therapist establish appropriate boundaries concerning treatment outcome responsibility by having him evaluate his treatment interventions and its results based on the principle that clinicians are responsible for input but not outcome, because clients have free will. Thus the therapist's knowledge, skills, and intervention strategies can be evaluated from a standard of best practices instead of what the client chooses to do with the intervention. Such strategies help clinicians manage their anxiety and feelings of anger and frustration.

How to Measure Change and Success

The long-term treatment goals for clients with multiple disorders take time to achieve, so it is important that agencies and clinicians use measures that help them identify the small steps that clients take toward these goals. Without these measures, clinicians cannot document or recognize important changes that clients are making and agencies cannot accurately measure their success rates. The lack of such information can lead to a sense of failure, burnout, or even funding reductions. Thus, supervisors need to expose clinicians to different models of change so they can clearly see and easily measure their clients' changes. Supervisors also need to take an active role in designing performance standards that meaningfully measure their agency's effectiveness. Chapter 10 presents several particularly useful measures for clients with co-occurring disorders that can be associated with performance standards.

Ensuring That Interactions Are Collegial

Usually numerous professionals provide services to the same client, bringing different levels of training, experience, and perspective on the focus of treatment. These differences always create the potential for interdisciplinary conflicts during collaboration or treatment coordination. Common areas of conflict include the following questions:

- Should the focus of treatment be on the mental health problem, the substance use problem, or some other aspect of treatment?
- Where should the client be treated?
- Does the usage indicate a substance dependence or a substance abuse disorder?
- Should abstinence be required or worked toward?
- How does one delineate between a mental disorder or a substance-induced disorder?
- Should usage result in removal from a program?
- Should medication be prescribed to someone still using alcohol or drugs?
- What medications should be prescribed?

The answers to these questions often vary depending on the client and the clinicians on the case, thus the supervisor must create a work atmosphere that is open to various viewpoints of others and open to examining one's own reactions to other views. To provide effective treatment for individuals with co-occurring disorders, a great deal of knowledge and skills must be integrated from a variety of professional disciplines and treatment models. Thus the professional differences encountered when addressing some of the previous issues must be framed by the supervisor as an opportunity to expand one's own knowledge and skill base, instead of as a power struggle. The supervisor can do this by emphasizing that no single discipline or profession has all the knowledge or skills to effectively address all the needs of this population. Supervisors can also promote this atmosphere by helping staff see how another treatment approach might be different, but the goal of that treatment is still the same as theirs. Finding this common ground can help keep the discussion between professionals focused on treatment techniques instead of philosophical or personal differences, thus greatly increasing their ability to find additional common ground.

Supervisors also need to attend to less than confident clinicians ("I do not know enough to give my input into the treatment plan") and overconfident clinicians ("I am more capable of helping this individual than others"). Both positions interfere with the development of collegial treatment relationships and can limit the treatment options available to clients. Supervisors must take a stand that the viewpoints of all professionals involved in the treatment of a client are of equal importance to the successful outcome of treatment. The supervisor needs to help the under-confident therapist accept his expertise and find the voice to express it. For another therapist, the intervention involves lowering the therapist's defenses enough to see that considering the options of others can only increase his or her clinical effectiveness.

Dealing with Ethical Concerns

Several ethical concerns often arise when clinicians work with individuals with co-occurring disorders; they involve personal sharing, physical contact, disclosure of information, and documentation of services. Some mental health professionals are trained to disclose virtually nothing about themselves, while many substance abuse professionals are themselves in recovery and are comfortable sharing that and other personal information. Likewise, when it comes to physical contact, most substance abuse professionals are used to being warm and familiar toward their clients; they consider it normal to touch a hand or shoulder or to close a session or group with a hug. In fact, substance abuse therapists who themselves are in recovery may encounter clients at self-help meetings. Mental health professionals, on the other hand, are often trained not to touch, but to teach clients to use words rather than actions to express themselves. Supervisors must help clinicians develop appropriate boundaries concerning sharing and touching that are based on whether particular actions would be helpful or disruptive for a particular client. For some clients appropriate sharing or touching by a therapist can promote a sense of security, affiliation, and hope that is helpful to the treatment process. However, for other clients such actions can create confusion about the therapeutic relationship. Because of the emotional or cognitive complications of their disorders, clients might interpret such behaviors as threatening, intrusive, or an invitation for a nonprofessional personal relationship. Depending on the training and professional orientation of a therapist and the clients in treatment, the supervisor may need to either promote appropriate sharing or touching or discourage such activities.

Difficulties concerning the disclosure of information usually occur because of misunderstandings of the different laws governing confidentiality and who is authorized to receive client information. Confidentiality regulations covering substance abuse treatment are some of the strictest in the nation. They are set by federal law (Federal Rules and Regulations on the Confidentiality of Alcohol and Drug Abuse Patient Records, 42 CFR Part 2) and are uniformly applied to all professionals providing substance abuse treatment. Mental health confidentiality laws are a combination of federal and state regulations. The substance abuse confidentially guidelines apply to treatment activities, not types of agencies providing services. Thus if therapists are providing substance abuse treatment in a mental health clinic, they must abide by substance abuse confidentiality regulations. Supervisors need to clearly define for their staff what confidentiality rules they must abide by and to whom they can disclose information. Two publications by the federal government's Center for Substance Abuse Treatment (CSAT) (1994b, 1999) offer excellent guidance in everyday language on how to comply with regulations. These are Technical Assistance Publication (TAP) Number 13, "Confidentiality of Patient Records for Alcohol and Other Drug Treatment," and TAP 24, "Welfare Reform and Substance Abuse Treatment Confidentiality: General Guidance for Reconciling Need to Know and Privacy."

Another ethical consideration that may challenge the therapist is the frequent and ongoing work with other agencies. If collaboration and cooperation exist, all is well. Many therapists run into barriers that limit the client's access to services at other agencies or the ability to succeed using those services. The therapist, in an attempt to advocate for the client, may fall into a demanding and angry mode of interaction with the other service providers. At such times, therapists may rationalize another professional's motives (such as stating that she is doing this because of issues with her own children) or question the quality of that program. Such behavior can disrupt the relationship between the two agencies in such a manner that future client referrals become even more difficult. Supervisors must be very proactive when their staff is having difficulties with referral agencies. They must help their staff clarify their issues in a nonpersonal way, express what they need from the other agency, and why they think the other agency can provide it. Supervisors need to emphasize to staff that they should not confront the other agency until they have these clarifications. Of course staff will need to vent about frustrations with individuals and rules; however, that should be kept only within the context of supervision. In many cases, the supervisor will need to address the problems and take the lead in discussing issues with the supervisor of the other agency. The key is to keep the discussion at the professional level between the staff of both agencies. Focus on treatment, not personal issues.

Finally, some clinicians are surprised to learn that treatment documentation is an ethical concern. Documentation is often the only means by which clinicians can demonstrate that they are using best practices to treat a client. It also documents that the treatment needs of each disorder are addressed and that clinicians have followed all local, state, and federal requirements concerning such issues as duty to warn, reporting suspected child or elder abuse, and maintaining client confidentiality. Clinicians often fail to effectively fulfill this essential clinical responsibility. Supervisors must set very clear guidelines for staff concerning what and when clinical information must be documented and then monitor that it is being done.

System Blending

Many treatment services for co-occurring disorders are collaborative efforts between substance abuse and mental health programs. Such collaborative efforts can result in a variety of supervisory configurations. Supervisors may find themselves supervising some staff for certain activities and other staff for other activities. Also, staff may receive additional supervision from other supervisors. Such supervisory situations have the potential to create confusion and conflicts over responsibilities and best clinical intervention for a specific situation.

For example, a substance abuse therapist is on loan ten hours a week to a mental health program to conduct substance abuse assessments and to co-lead two groups with a mental health therapist for clients with co-occurring disorders. The substance abuse therapist finds himself in a dual supervision situation. The supervision of his treatment activities at the substance abuse treatment program is unchanged, but a mental health supervisor now supervises his activities at the mental health program. During a substance abuse assessment at the mental health program, a client who has bipolar and alcohol dependence disorders and a history of misusing her medication refuses to sign a release that would allow the substance abuse therapist to talk with her private doctor. The substance abuse therapist, who is used to denying services to clients who refuse to sign such releases, brings the situation to the attention of his mental health supervisor. Instead of receiving support for his position, he is advised to work on building more trust in the therapeutic relationship so that the client will be willing to sign the release. When he tells his substance abuse supervisor about this, the supervisor states that such a suggestion prevents the doctor from knowing about her alcohol dependence disorder and enables her to continue misusing her medication. Thus the clinician ends up receiving conflicting supervisory advice and begins to believe that his substance abuse work at the mental health program will fail because its standard practices may be less than helpful.

Supervisors involved in collaborative treatment activities must work closely together and develop clear guidelines concerning supervisory responsibility. Furthermore, each supervisor must become familiar with the treatment philosophies, policies and procedures, standard treatment practices, and the politics that create the work environments of clinical staff. Such knowledge and awareness will help supervisors reduce potentially confusing or contradicting treatment recommendations; better understand why a therapist from another agency might choose a particular treatment approach; and help staff going into a new clinical setting understand why situations may be handled differently.

In the previous example, had the supervisors spent time together prior to the implementation of this collaborative effort, they could have developed guidelines concerning supervisory responsibilities and increased their understanding of each other's treatment system. They probably would have also developed a process for resolving clinical differences. The mental health supervisor would also have had a better understanding of the importance of setting limits concerning potential drug use, and the substance abuse therapist and supervisor would have had a better understanding of the importance of keeping an individual with a major mental disorder in treatment. Thus instead of developing warring camps, the supervisors could have focused on how to gain contact with the doctor and still keep the client in treatment.

SUPERVISORY SUPPORTS

Not only does the clinical staff need supervision, but so do clinical supervisors. Many clinical supervisors receive little if any oversight of their supervision. This is the result of several factors: clinical supervisors tend to be seasoned, thus the perception exists that they do not need supervision; the individual supervising the supervisor may not have a clinical background; and, depending on the size of the program, he or she may be the only clinical supervisor in the agency. Even though in most cases clinical supervisors are seasoned clinicians, it is highly unlikely they have extensive experience in providing supervision for staff treating individuals with co-occurring disorders. Programs treating this population must establish an oversight of supervision process for clinical supervisors.

As is true for the supervisory process for clinicians, this supervisory process must include formal, informal, and ongoing training components. This process can be established in a number of ways. Programs that have more than one clinical supervisor can establish formal meetings for this purpose. These meetings might be peer run or facilitated by a head supervisor, depending on the organizational structure of the program. When a program has just a single clinical supervisor and no one in the organization capable of providing the necessary supervision, a consultant can be hired to perform this task, arrangements can be made with another agency for this individual to participate in supervisory activities, or support can be given to that individual's participation in a community supervisory support group formed for such a purpose. Seasoned clinicians usually have peers with whom they have long histories and trusting relationships, and can turn to them to discuss supervisory difficulties that they are experiencing. It is important that clinical supervisors be encouraged and allowed to use these informal networks as long as client and personnel confidentiality rules are followed. Since the state-of-the-art treatment concerning this population is constantly expanding, it is also important that clinical supervisors regularly attend training sessions concerning the treatment of this population and other specific training targeted toward improving supervisory skills. Being continually faced with all the issues that need immediate attention, it is often easy for the management of treatment programs for co-occurring disorders to put the establishment of a supervision of supervision process low on the priority list. However, failure to establish such a process will reduce the overall quality of supervision clinicians receive and minimize the effectiveness of their clinical services.

CONCLUSION

The art of supervision will always be part intuition and part technique. In addition, the amount and type of supervision staff members need vary depending on knowledge and skill level, experience, and temperament of that clinician. As with clinicians, supervisors need to have specific qualities to be effective. This chapter reviewed those qualities, methods of establishing effective supervisory structures, common supervisory issues that arise during the treatment of individuals with co-occurring disorders, and how the clinical supervisors can also obtain supervision of their supervision. The next chapter focuses on the issues that program managers of these services must deal with on a day-to-day basis.

Chapter 8

Day-to-Day Program Management

Probably the most tedious, but absolutely the most important aspect of providing co-occurring disorders treatment services is the day-to-day management of these services. These management activities include the following:

- ensuring all information needed by funding sources is provided accurately and on time;
- developing and maintaining systems that ensure clients move through the treatment services in the easiest manner;
- developing and managing client and other data systems;
- ensuring compliance with all licensure requirements;
- developing and updating policies and procedures for all program activities; and
- maintaining effective working relations with other community agencies.

How and who performs these duties will often depend on the size of the program providing the services. In larger programs, each of these duties may be performed by a different individual, while in smaller programs one person may be responsible for several of these functions. Smaller programs require managers who can balance multiple tasks and accurately determine which tasks are most critical at any given time. Larger programs need managers who are willing to stay within the specific boundaries of their management tasks and who can hire competent individuals to which they delegate critical tasks. This chapter focuses on the issues that managers of co-occurring disorders treatment programs face when carrying out their management tasks.

QUALITIES OF AN EFFECTIVE MANAGER

The program manager has ultimate oversight and responsibility for the management, administrative, and clinical functions of a program that provides co-occurring disorders treatment services. In larger programs this job is normally the sole function of a single individual; in smaller programs this may be but one of many functions that this individual performs. In smaller programs the program manager might also perform clinical supervision functions; carry a caseload; or perform some of the administrative functions such as collecting data or writing and submitting required reports. However, regardless of the size of the program, ultimately one individual is responsible for answering to the community about how well these three functions are performed.

To be effective, individuals who perform this role need to possess certain qualities. These qualities include the following:

- the ability to exercise leadership;
- the ability to ensure the survival of the program;
- having an understanding of the traditions, values, and ethics that clinicians and administrative staff follow;
- being able to listen and consider all staff input while being decisive when necessary;
- the ability to communicate to all staff in a clear and timely manner the decisions made and the rationale for them;
- the ability to successfully develop relationships with other community agencies; and
- the ability to operate both as an ally and the loyal opposition when dealing with organizations that have authority over the program.

Although these are the qualities of any good mental health or substance abuse treatment program manager, they are also required of managers of co-occurring disorders treatment programs. The following is a description of these seven qualities and how they are used in the management of larger and smaller co-occurring disorders treatment services.

Leadership

As in the case of clinical supervision, leadership also plays an important part in the role of an effective manager of co-occurring disorders treatment services. However, except in very small programs in which the manager also functions as the clinical supervisor, the total focus of leadership in this role is to create an atmosphere of stability, ensuring that the staff have all the tools necessary to accomplish the program's mission, and inspiring them to accomplish this mission. To be effective, staff must work in a stable environment and be secure in their jobs. The staff must also believe that the program supports their work, which means having the proper tools available to them (such as adequate treatment space, availability of medication services, or availability of testing for client drug use). The final aspect of leadership at the managerial level involves promoting a belief among the staff and the community that the program is effective and contributes to the well-being of the community. In programs in which managers are clinical supervisors they must also perform the leadership functions of a clinical supervisor as outlined in Chapter 7, which can be a delicate balancing act.

Ensuring Program Survival

Although a clinical supervisor must be the advocate for effective clinical services, the manager must be an effective advocate for program survival. Program survival involves ensuring that the clinical services are being effectively provided and all necessary administrative and political tasks are attended to in a timely manner. Administrative and political tasks include the following:

- meeting licensure requirements;
- timely submission of budgets or reimbursement requests;
- submitting accurate data requirements to funding and other monitoring agencies;
- properly processing employee time sheets so checks are available on time; and
- promptly responding to such issues as human rights complaints, advocacy groups' information requests, or speaker requests from community organizations.

As is true for the clinical supervisor, the manager must at times choose between clinical and program survival needs. To effectively fulfill the manager's role, this individual must always be the advocate of the program survival needs in those instances. In smaller programs in which the manager and the clinical supervisor is often the same person, that individual must have the capacity to accurately determine if the clinical or administrative needs of the program are the most critical to its survival at any given time. In larger programs, the manager's role is always to advocate for the completion of administrative requirements.

Knowledge of Staff Traditions, Values, and Ethics

Managers must be knowledgeable in the traditions, values, and ethics of the clinical and administrative staff working for the program. A program providing co-occurring disorders treatment may have staff whose professional identities are as doctors, nurses, social workers, substance abuse counselors, family therapists, case managers, computer specialists, medical records technicians, financial managers, administrative assistants, or receptionists. Although it is highly unlikely that a manager will have had personal experience providing each of the functions, it is possible for the manager to be aware of the traditions, values, and ethics attached to these professional identities. Without this knowledge, managers may attempt to resolve problems or introduce policies and procedures in a manner that will run counter to certain traditions, values, and ethics and thus his or her policies will be resisted or not carried out by portions of the staff. When this occurs, clients receive inconsistent treatment and tension and conflict develop among staff members, which results in reduced program performance. Managers not fully aware of the traditions, values, and ethics of all their staff members must always solicit input from them concerning proposed changes in program services or procedures. In smaller programs in which staff often perform multiple tasks and supervisory layers are limited, this input normally can be obtained faster than in larger programs with multiple layers of supervision and highly specialized staff. Hence major program changes can usually be accomplished much faster in smaller programs than in larger ones.

Being Decisive While Listening to Staff Imput

As discussed in Chapter 5, many co-occurring disorders treatment services are in the initial stages of their development and thus are evolving treatment philosophies and practices, clarifying decisions concerning who they can treat effectively, and establishing long-term working relationships with many other community organizations. Even established co-occurring disorders treatment programs make frequent changes in practices and procedures because of the rapidly evolving knowledge base concerning treatment of these disorders. During this change process multiple decisions normally need to be made. Staff needs to know that the manager will listen to what they say, that their input is valued, and that when a decision is needed, it will be made. Staff members who know that they are genuinely listened to and have input into program decisions will develop ownership of a program's activities. Staff members who also know that a decision will be made when it is necessary will develop a sense of security by knowing that they are not on a rudderless ship. Both of these management actions are at different ends of the same decision-making process and require a manager who can use both democratic and enlightened monarch management styles. Effective managers know when to use each style. Since input is strongly related to access, managers of larger programs must work harder at soliciting staff input than managers of smaller programs. Larger programs normally have two or more layers of supervision between line staff and the manager while in smaller programs all staff normally have direct access to the manager.

Communicating Decisions in a Clear and Timely Manner

Because co-occurring disorders treatment programs are constantly evolving, many decisions that affect how staff perform their jobs must be communicated to them by the manager. Once a decision has been made, staff will need to know in a timely manner exactly what that decision is and why it was made. Staff do not necessarily need to agree with a decision, but they are much more likely to abide by it if they understand the rationale behind it. The manager's style or the importance of the decision will often dictate how the information is communicated. Some managers are uncomfortable in communicating face to face with large groups so they will send the information by memo, voice mail, or e-mail. Other managers prefer meeting directly with the staff to share this information. In general, the style is not as important as that it is done in a clear and timely manner, but there are a few exceptions. A decision involving a major policy change that will result in staff needing to express a great number of thoughts and feelings is best presented to all staff in a large group. In smaller programs in which all staff report to the manager and all staff have regular contact with one another, the norm would be to communicate face to face. In larger programs that have multiple supervisory layers, the importance of the decision often dictates how it is communicated. Again, the timeliness and clarity of the message is more important than the manner it which it is presented.

Working Effectively with Other Community Organizations

In order to survive, a program must receive support from a variety of community organizations. Some of these organizations refer clients to the program; some provide essential support services for the program's clients; and some serve as advocates for the continuation of the program. As is true for the staff, each of these community organizations has a wide range of traditions, values, and ethics. Program managers must have the ability to be aware of these differences, learn the language of these organizations, and maintain friendly relationships when dealing with organizations that operate in different ways or have different community viewpoints. For example, a substance abuse advocacy organization in the community might not believe medication should be provided to clients until they have had thirty days of sobriety, which is counter to the medication-prescribing policy of a co-occurring disorders treatment program. The co-occurring disorders treatment program's manager can choose to engage in a heated debate with that advocacy group in an attempt to win the argument, or can choose to listen to what they have to say, develop an understanding of why they have taken this position, examine the clinical rationale of the program's medicating policy, and agree to disagree. The latter action acknowledges differences but still allows the program and the advocacy group to work together on issues in which they are in agreement, thus maintaining that important relationship. More detailed discussions of these types of relationships are presented in Chapters 9 and 10. Smaller programs tend to be found in smaller communities with fewer community groups with which to maintain relationships; however, community organizations tend to be dominated by individuals with strong personalities. Thus managers of smaller programs need to have the ability to interface effectively with individuals who have very strong and set opinions. Managers of larger programs, which tend to be located in larger communities, need to be able to interact effectively with multiple organizations that often have large numbers of staff or members and whose methods of interaction tend to be more formal.

Working Effectively with Authorizing and Monitoring Organizations

All co-occurring disorders treatment programs have organizations that authorize them to legally provide their services and monitor their performance. These organizations range from licensing or certifying bodies to community advisory groups. To be effective, managers must be able to interact with these organizations at times as an ally and at times as part of the loyal opposition. In smaller programs, the manager may be the primary person who interacts with each of these agencies; in larger programs, administrative staff do most of the interaction while the manager monitors the effectiveness of this interaction. Detailed descriptions of interactions with these types of organizations are presented in a later section of this chapter and in Chapters 9 and 10.

DEVELOPING THE NECESSARY MANAGEMENT TOOLS (POLICIES AND PROCEDURES)

Many new mental health or substance abuse clinicians have spent the first few days at their new job reading the agency's policy and procedure manual. Though the feeling most associated with this image is somewhere in the rage of deadly boring, if such a manual does not exist then a program has no way to guarantee equal treatment of clients and staff and runs the risk of increased liability. Boring as it is, the policy and procedures manual provides managers with the standards by which they can monitor the clinical, personnel, and administrative functions of the program. Policy and procedures manuals lay out who will be provided treatment services; what these services will be; what is expected from the staff and what the staff's rights are; what data is to be collected; how the data is to be collected; and what will be done with it after it is collected. In larger programs the manager will often delegate writing of specific policies to other staff and will function more as an approving agent than a creator of procedure. In smaller programs the manager is usually very involved in creating policies by either writing them directly or being part of a staff group that creates them. Either way, it is still the manager's responsibility to see that all activities of the treatment program have written policies and procedures which provide guidance concerning how they should be carried out. This section will discuss specific policies and procedures that managers of co-occurring disorders treatment programs should ensure are included in their manuals.

Treatment Policies and Procedures

These policies and procedures provide guidance concerning who will be treated, how individuals can access treatment, what is involved in the treatment process, and how treatment may be ended. Four areas in this client flow process require guidance in the form of policies and procedures. These are eligibility, admission, treatment, and discharge or referral. Eligibility covers who the program is to provide services for, and information concerning this is usually found both in the program's mission statement and its policies and procedures manual. Program managers must ensure that their mission statement includes the program's responsibility to provide co-occurring disorders treatment and that the admission criteria clearly spell out which subgroups of individuals with co-occurring disorders the program is designed to treat (see Chapter 3 for a description of co-occurring disorders subgroups). When a mission statement is a broad overview of a program's purpose, the admission criteria must be very specific. For example, a program's mission statement might include a statement indicating that a program will provide treatment for individuals with co-occurring disorders; however, its admission criteria indicate that it treats individuals with less serious psychiatric symptoms who also have substance use disorders. Since most co-occurring disorders treatment programs will not provide services to all four subgroups of this population, policies and procedures must also include a description of actions that will be taken when a client does not meet the admission criteria.

The next area that policies and procedures must address is clients' points of entry—where and how clients can access services. Some programs have a single point of entry (a phone number to call and ask for an appointment) and some programs have multiple points of entry (a phone number that can be called to ask for an appointment, an outreach worker who can set up an appointment, and a walk-in center whose staff can also set up an appointment). Managers of programs that serve individuals with and without co-occurring disorders must decide if all their points of entry are to be used for individuals with co-occurring disorders or if just certain points of entry are appropriate. Many individuals with co-occurring disorders have ambivalent feelings about entering treatment and/or have limited social skills. Thus it must be ensured that the requirements to access services at any point of entry for individuals with co-occurring disorders be limited and that services be offered in a very timely manner. Smaller programs tend to have single points of entry and fewer requirements for admission than larger programs.

Treatment policies and procedures must also cover specific practices that must be followed during a client's course of treatment. In smaller programs that provide only one set of services (such as outpatient treatment) the policies and procedures usually cover such issues as type of services to be offered, length of treatment, participation requirements, etc.; larger programs that offer several components of the continuum of care must also develop policies and procedures addressing when and how a client can move from one part of the treatment continuum to another. The issues that must be addressed in this portion of the policies and procedures manual involve ensuring that clients receive the level and types of services they need and what action the agency will take if a specific type or level of service is not available. For example, a policy may state that any client exhibiting psychiatric symptoms must receive an evaluation for medication or any client who is unable to maintain abstinence must be evaluated for residential treatment. Such policies provide the manager with criteria for determining if a staff member is following accepted treatment practices for this population. Likewise, many communities do not have full continuum of services for individuals with co-occurring disorders, so policies and procedures need to be in place that outline staff members' actions when a client needs a level of service that is unavailable in the community. It may be the policy of a program that individuals with co-occurring disorders in need of residential treatment will be provided outpatient, crisis intervention, and detoxification services when residential treatment services are unavailable. Again, this allows a manager to determine if staff members are providing the level of treatment that is closest to the needs of a client.

Finally, policies and procedures must be developed concerning how a client is to be discharged from treatment or referred out to another program. Managers of programs that treat multiple subgroups of the co-occurring disorders population or who treat individuals both with and without co-occurring disorders must ensure that their policies and procedures concerning discharge and referral are specific to each subgroup population. An appropriate discharge criterion for a high-functioning client without a co-occurring disorder, such as failing to attend treatment regularly, would not necessarily be an appropriate discharge criterion for an individual with a substance use and psychotic disorder. Likewise, how an individual is referred for other services will vary among clients. The procedures for higher-functioning clients might involve providing clients with the information about how to set up an appointment; the procedures for referring lower-functioning clients might include setting up the appointment for them, transporting them to the appointment, or helping them fill out all the necessary admission forms. Again, it is important for programs serving different populations to have discharge and referral policies and procedures that reflect the skills and capabilities of all their clients. Smaller programs will normally serve fewer treatment populations; larger programs will usually have a greater variety of treatment populations.

Personnel Policies and Procedures

Many managers believe that 90 percent of personnel time is spent on 10 percent of the personnel. This number may be a bit high, but it probably accurately describes the emotional process that managers experience when dealing with difficult personnel issues. Personnel policies and procedures are put into place to help manage these emotional situations by clearly defining acceptable and unacceptable employee behavior. These policies and procedures normally range from work attendance to paperwork compliance and involve such issues as job descriptions, key elements of performance, or general personnel regulations. No policy and procedure manual can cover every personnel issue, but it can cover those which occur most commonly. The personnel issues that most frequently arise in programs providing co-occurring disorders treatment services are staff skill levels, staff training, staff relations with other staff and other professionals in the community, and staff treatment of clients.

Many clinicians providing co-occurring disorders treatment services will need to acquire much of their knowledge and develop many of their skills on the job, thus clear personnel policies and procedures need to be developed regarding the knowledge and skills needed and the timeline for acquiring them. An employee job description might require an individual to have or obtain a substance abuse and mental health treatment certification or license within two years of employment. This would ensure that staff members have a basic knowledge and skill level for dealing with both mental health and substance use issues. In another scenario, a job description might also state specific skills and knowledge that an employee must be able to demonstrate within a year (specific knowledge and skills needed to effectively treat individuals with co-occurring disorders are found in Chapter 6 of this book). The key is to have a policy that requires staff to demonstrate some level of efficiency in treating individuals with co-occurring disorders. Attached to this policy must be a set of procedures that outlines how this efficiency is measured and what actions will be taken if a staff member fails to achieve the required level of performance. In the first example, efficiency is documented by licensure or certification; the second example requires standardization of supervisory observation or some form of testing. The latter is more complicated to administer; however, it will provide a truer measure of competency. When establishing these procedures, program management must consider the capacity to actually carry them out. Smaller programs must rely more on external measures; larger programs may have the management and supervisory staff to conduct their own measurements. The final part of the procedures is to clearly state the consequences for failing to achieve a specific level of efficiency. This can range from dismissal to the development of a training plan. Usually it is best to have a procedure that allows managers a flexible response. One employee who is doing a good job but is having some difficulty passing a licensure exam could be given a time extension; another employee who is not doing a good job would not be given a time extension.

Another important part of this section of the policies and procedures manual concerns staff training requirements. Not only do most staff need to acquire co-occurring disorders treatment knowledge and skills, but even staff who have high efficiency in this area need to attend training regularly if they are to keep abreast of the rapidly expanding knowledge about co-occurring disorders. Thus, specific policies and procedures are needed concerning staff training requirements that include the amount and type of training staff must attend and how this training will be documented. The key is to ensure that a program has a policy concerning expected staff knowledge and skills that includes training requirements for treating co-occurring disorders and a procedure for measuring this efficiency.

Clients with co-occurring disorders need multiple treatment services, thus staff providing treatment services must maintain effective working relationships with other professionals both within and without the agency. Staff who are unable to develop such effective working relationships will be unable to coordinate their treatment activities with staff who provide other treatments or will be unable to access needed support services for their clients from other community agencies. Thus it is important to include such skills into written job expectations and have policies and procedures in place that allow for the measurement of these skills and methods for addressing deficiencies when identified. Measurable methods can range from documentation in the personnel record of complaints received or deficiencies observed to formalized evaluations by other professionals working with agency staff members. Larger programs usually have greater resources and thus can quantitatively document a staff member's ability to develop effective working relationships; in smaller programs the manager often has hands-on experience with all of the staffs' ability to develop such relationships. Staff treatment of clients usually is covered in detail by human rights laws (see page 163 of this chapter); however it is important to include in any written policy expectations that staff working with individuals with co-occurring disorders must address their mental health and substance abuse treatment issues in an integrated manner. Clinical staff that cannot provide integrated treatment cannot be effective with this treatment population. Including the previously mentioned criteria into an agency's policies and procedures ensures that the most commonly arising personnel issues can be addressed.

Administrative Policies and Procedures

All program personnel need to know the diagnostic and demographic characteristics of their clients and must report certain data elements about their treatment activities. This information includes such items as: age, sex, and race of clients being served; types of disorders that need to be treated; and number of clients served, number of services provided, or the number of days in treatment. Information collected by a program is usually dictated by internal needs and outside requirements. All program managers perceive the need to collect certain pieces of information to ascertain if the program is effectively performing its functions. They also need to ensure that the information is collected that is needed to meet all reporting requirements to outside agencies, such as those providing funding or licensure. Some of the information collected is used both internally and externally; other pieces of information are used just internally or externally. Many programs now use computers to store essential information, but in almost all cases, a paper-tracking system coexists with computer databases. Obviously computers are much more efficient at storing and analyzing large sets of data than are paper and pencil methods, however, some data elements are just too small or complex to work well with a computer system. Most program managers feel they are often drowning in data collection and reporting requirements. The purpose of this section is not to discuss ways to lessen this burden, because it will probably only get worse, but to present the data elements that programs must collect in order to monitor the effectiveness of co-occurring disorders treatment services.

Several specific data elements are needed to monitor the nature of clients with co-occurring disorders being serviced, as well as the effectiveness of the services provided them. These data elements are the ability to identify all clients' diagnoses; a functioning level measure; time between request for service and first services; number of clients remaining in treatment at least ninety days (see outcome measures in Chapter 10); number of clients in need of more intensive services than are being provided; and to what other programs clients are referred. Having this information available, the management team of a co-occurring disorders treatment program will know exactly the types of clients being served, how accessible the treatment services are, the program's ability to retain clients in treatment, and if its clients are receiving the level of treatment services necessary. This knowledge allows the management team to evaluate if it is fulfilling its mission to treat a specific subgroup of this population, how accessible and effective treatment services are, and if clients in need of more intensive services are being connected with them, or if a strategic plan needs to be developed concerning how to create those services. Each of the above requirements is essential to answer these questions.

MAINTAINING EFFECTIVE RELATIONSHIPS WITH MONITORING ORGANIZATIONS

Every program has oversight groups that authorize its existence or monitors its performance. At a minimum, these oversight organizations include licensing or certifying bodies that authorize the program to provide services or endorse their quality; an agency that provides funding for the services; an agency that is responsible for monitoring if the treatment program is respecting the human rights of its clients; and usually a community group that has been appointed to provide oversight or advisory duties to the program. It is the manager's responsibility to maintain effective working relationships with these various monitoring groups. This section discusses the nature of these relationships and examines common issues that arise when co-occurring disorders treatment services are provided.

Licensing and Certifying Bodies

These organizations either authorize the program to legally provide these services or certify that the program meets some basic quality level. Managers must be familiar with the rules and procedures that must be followed to meet the requirements of these organizations. In larger programs the direct contact with these organizations is usually by an administrative staff member; the function of the manager in that instance is to supervise the activities of that staff member.

In smaller programs the manager is usually the primary individual who interacts with licensing and certifying bodies. The most common issues that managers of co-occurring disorder programs encounter are duplicate licensure or certifying requirements, compliance with regulations or required operating procedures that in no way contribute to quality co-occurring disorders treatment services, and regulations or required operating procedures that actually are contrary to effective co-occurring disorders treatment practices.

For example, a program operates in a state that has licensing regulations for mental health and substance abuse treatment services but not for co-occurring disorders treatment. If a program is to provide co-occurring treatment services, it must be licensed to provide both mental health and substance abuse treatment. This duplicate licensing process is very time-consuming for the treatment program. It requires meeting two sets of regulations and having two agencies make formal and informal visitations and inspections. In some instances the same regulated action (such as when treatment plans are developed) will have different requirements (such as one licensing agency requiring an initial treatment plan be developed at intake and the other licensing agency requiring that a treatment plan be developed within the first thirty days of treatment). This results in the program's leaders having to choose which requirement to follow and then having to document with the other licensing agency why it is not following their requirement. Also, inspectors from these two licensing agencies might interpret the same regulation in different ways, resulting in confusion concerning how to meet the regulations or having to comply with the regulation in a duplicate manner.

In another example, a co-occurring disorders program is required by a state mental health licensing agency to document its activities in helping clients obtain Social Security disability benefits. This documentation includes data collection, the creation of policies and procedures, and follow-up activities. Since many clients in traditional mental health services are eligible for these benefits, this documentation makes good sense in the context of mental health services. However, the co-occurring disorders treatment program is designed to serve only clients in Subgroup III (high substance abuse symptoms and low psychiatric symptoms) and thus it is rare for a client to be eligible for Social Security disability.

In still another example, a co-occurring disorders program must be certified by a specific national certifying body to be eligible for Medicaid funding. The certifying body requires that clients be involved in the development of their treatment plans and agree with all aspects of it to meet particular certifying requirements. Many clients entering the treatment program are still in denial about either their substance use or mental disorders, therefore this certifying requirement makes it very difficult to address these issues without the clients' permission. Such requirements are contrary to accepted treatment practices for individuals with co-occurring disorders. Managers of co-occurring disorders treatment programs must be able to meet multiple licensing and certifying requirements while being able to clearly articulate with licensing and certifying bodies why their program should be exempted from current regulations and other requirements that place undue burdens on their operations or contradict effective co-occurring treatment services.

Funding Sources

Organizations that fund a program's treatment services will want to know that their funds are wisely spent and result in effective treatment. Thus the manager must ensure that appropriate accounting procedures are followed, that funds are used in the manner in which they were intended, and expected results are obtained. Smaller programs will usually need to contract out the accounting activities to a professional accounting firm because they normally will not have the expertise to conduct these activities or have the administrative or management time to dedicate to them. Larger programs usually have at least one administrative staff member who provides this function. Ensuring that funds are spent as they were intended can sometimes become a bit vague. Almost all funding sources require the submission of a detailed budget with line items spelling out how much can be spent on each activity; however, line items always leave some room for interpretation. Both the funding source and treatment program may agree that $5,000 can be spent for staff training. However, what constitutes appropriate training for staff providing co-occurring disorders treatment services may be viewed differently by the funding source officials and the treatment program administrators.

Likewise, a line item funding security deposits for clients in a co-occurring disorders treatment program providing services for homeless individuals might result in different viewpoints concerning what constitutes a security deposit. Differing interpretations will occur from time to time; the key is for the manager to be willing to dialogue with the funding agency about these differences both before and after funds are expended and be able to make the case why spending funds in a specific manner will have a positive impact on clinical services. Chapter 10 examines in detail performance and outcome measures that can be used to demonstrate the program's effectiveness, and an effective manager must also ensure that the program is following appropriate accounting procedures. Should a manager fail to perform these tasks effectively, the program runs the risk of losing the funds it needs to operate its services.

Human Rights Monitoring Organizations

All programs must adhere to a set of human rights laws that describe how clients may be treated while receiving services. These laws usually cover what rights clients have in the treatment process; how clients can file complaints when they believe their rights have been violated; how these compliants must be investigated; and what consequences should be imposed if it is found that clients' rights have been violated. Programs providing co-occurring disorders treatment blend substance abuse and mental health treatment practices, so it is not uncommon for clients previously treated in a traditional substance abuse or mental health setting to question some of the practices they encounter when entering a co-occurring disorders treatment program.

Clients with mental health treatment backgrounds might wonder if the requirement to provide urine samples is a violation of their rights. Clients with a substance abuse treatment background might wonder if the requirement to take medication as prescribed by the program's psychiatrist is a violation of their rights. Although these are standard treatment practices in a co-occurring disorders treatment program, they may be new and alien to clients coming from another treatment background. Thus it is quite possible that a co-occurring disorders treatment program will experience human rights complaints on a regular basis.

In addition, when co-occurring disorders treatment services are new to a community, the agency tasked with investigating human rights violations will also frequently be unaware of common treatment practices for this population and the clinical rationales behind them. Program managers must be fully aware of the human rights regulations governing their program's treatment activities; ensure that clients have access to literature or staff who can explain how the program treatment requirements are in compliance with the human rights laws; and establish a dialogue with the monitoring agency for the purpose of informing them of current clinical practices and the rationale for them. This relationship should also include requesting a consultation to interpret vague regulations. Such actions will help minimize the number of human rights complaints with which the program must contend (often involving a great deal of staff time); ensure that the monitoring agency fully understands why the program uses certain clinical practices; and ensure that the program position will be clearly understood when complaints are filed. Program size usually does not play a significant part in the management of this relationship.

Advisory and Oversight Boards

Advisory and oversight boards are organizations that are normally found on a program's organizational chart and generally are composed of community professionals and citizens who are invested in what the program is attempting to achieve. These individuals are often also active in other related advocacy groups in the community. The amount of real authority these organizations have will vary significantly between programs. In some instances, consent is needed from these organizations before a program can take certain actions, and in other instances they serve solely in an advisory capacity. Regardless of the group's level of authority, it can be a powerful ally in promoting expanded program resources or resisting program cuts. Effective managers cultivate the power of these groups by including them in all major decisions, keeping them informed about major issues being faced by the program, and providing them with the information needed to be an effective lobbying group for the interests of the program. In smaller communities such advisory or oversight boards are often the only advocacy group for a program's services in the community. Even in larger communities, services for individuals with co-occurring disorders are usually the new kid on the block, and thus do not have well-established advocacy groups in the community. Failure to maintain an effective working relationship with these groups can either block the authorization or implementation of important program activities or undermine the essential political support needed from the community to ensure program survive.

CONCLUSION

This chapter discussed the issues involved in the day-to-day management of treatment programs providing services for individuals with co-occurring disorders and what tools managers need to effectively manage such programs. It presented qualities that managers of such programs must possess, specific issues that need to be addressed in any policy and procedures manual of a program providing co-occurring disorders, and issues involved in maintaining effective working relationships with organizations that monitored the activities of co-occurring disorders treatment programs. Also discussed was how the size of a program affects these issues. The next chapter discusses issues involved in operating a co-occurring disorders treatment program in a multilevel/multi-organization system.

Chapter 9

Operating Within a Larger System

Every program that provides treatment services for individuals with co-occurring disorders operates within a larger system. The larger system is usually a mix of public and private organizations that operate from viewpoints that derive from national, state, or local perspectives. This multilevel/multi-organization system includes organizations that the treatment program reports to; organizations that provide essential treatment and support services to the program's clients; and at times organizations that report to the treatment program. At any given time a co-occurring disorder treatment program may have to maintain effective relationships with oversight organizations, collegial organizations providing essential treatment and support services to its clients, and organizations or treatment components it oversees. The nature of relationships in such multilevel/multi-organization systems are complex and follow many of the tenets of general System Theory proposed by von Bertalanffy (1968). This chapter will focus on the nature of systems providing services to individuals with co-occurring disorders and the common types of relationships that organizations have in these systems.

NATURE OF MULTILEVEL/ MULTI-ORGANIZATIONAL SYSTEMS

At a minimum, multilevel/multi-organization systems involved in co-occurring disorders treatment are usually composed of federal, state, local, and sometimes private funding sources; mental health, substance abuse, and possibly stand-alone co-occurring disorders treatment providers; organizations that refer clients; organizations that provide essential client support services; and licensing and certifying bodies. Such systems have six common characteristics.

- They are composed of organizations that have mutual and conflicting needs.
- Interactions between the organizations are formal and informal.
- The nature of the interactions between organizations are based on the history between the organizations.
- Traditions and certain mutually accepted ways of communicating within this system must be followed.
- Power within the system is based on a mixture of hierarchical structure, funding flow, community support, and personal charisma.
- The system will resist any substantial change.

The key to developing effective relationships in multilevel/multi-organization systems is in accepting how organizations operate and in developing flexible responses to these six traits.

A program that provides co-occurring disorders treatment services has the same need as its funding source, its authorizing body, and its referral sources, which is to ensure that effective treatment services are provided for individuals with co-occurring disorders. However, whereas the program's primary focus centers on ensuring effective treatment services, other agencies primarily focus on the receipt of data that demonstrates the program's effectiveness. Hence there are congruent and conflicting needs among these organizations. The program must be organized in a manner that allows allocation of sufficient resources to accomplish both tasks. For example, if program directors do not hire sufficient administrative staff or invest in an adequate computer system then the data needed for reports to oversight agencies must be compiled by the clinical and management staff. All clinical and management staff will perform some administrative tasks; however, if too much of their time is absorbed in this function the clinical and management activities of the program will suffer, causing the program to lose status in the system. Likewise, if reports to oversight organizations are inaccurate or not submitted in a timely manner, the program's relationship with these organizations will suffer. To operate effectively in a multilevel/multi-organizational system a program must ensure that all these tasks are performed well.

All organizations in such systems have both formal and informal communication channels. Formal communication channels include regular meetings between the organizations' staff, reports that provide specific types of information on a regular basis, or specific procedures for resolving problems between the organizations. Informal communication channels result from personal relationships developed among the staff members of these organizations and usually occur on an as-needed basis. Both are essential in forming a good working relationship between the organizations; however, it is important that one communication channel does not undermine or replace the other.

For example, a co-occurring disorders outpatient treatment program has an ongoing relationship with the local parole and probation office that refers numerous individuals for services. Set procedures exist for referring clients for services and reporting on treatment status or progress. The managers of both organizations met three times a year to discuss any issues or trends. The clinicians and the probation and parole officers also meet once a year for a joint training. In addition to these formal processes, many personal relationships between the line staff of these two organizations have formed as a result of sharing many clients over the years. In this instance, many of the day-to-day issues between these organizations can be resolved through informal communication channels, while for larger programmatic or philosophical issues formal methods of resolution are found at both the management and staff levels.

All organizations in a system have a history with one another. All communications are based on some current need, but they always occur within the context of past communications. Agencies with histories of good working relationships tend to have more open and impromptu communications; agencies with a history of adversarial relationships tend to have guarded and formalized communications. Since open and impromptu communication is usually more productive, agencies operating in a system will need to maintain their good working relationships and attempt to create a new history with agencies with which they have had an adversarial relationship in the past. A residential co-occurring disorders treatment program has a good working relationship with the local public detoxification program that regularly refers clients to the residential program; in the past, the treatment program had an adversarial relationship with a private agency that operates several counselor-monitored group homes. The adversarial relationship evolved from competition between these two agencies regarding several local funding initiatives. Although communication patterns are free flowing between the residential and the detoxification program that facilitates client placement, the communication patterns between the residential and the group home programs are often tense and very formalized. The private agency accepts some clients of the residential program, but the referral process is very tedious and rigid. Referral forms are extensive, little direct communication exists between referring staff members and the admission counselor, and a client's entry is often delayed because of minor paperwork mistakes. Also, some clients are denied admission because the private program management does not trust the accuracy of the residential program staff's evaluation of a client's stability.

A new history between these two organizations might be created in several ways. The residential program administrator might approach the private agency administrator and acknowledge that issues between the programs may be affecting client treatment and suggest that a private consultant be brought in to help them work out their differences. Both organizations could come together and jointly submit proposals for local or federal funding and then share any received funds. Also, the managers of the two programs might begin meeting regularly in an attempt to ameliorate their differences.

Familiar interaction patterns create comfort and normally facilitate communications. Thus, a multilevel/multi-organization system will create traditions and mutually agreed-upon ways of communicating and interacting. These include such issues as who can talk to whom; how this communication can occur; when and in what format it must occur; or what can and cannot be addressed.

Sometimes a tradition or a method of interaction no longer fits the personalities involved or outlives its usefulness and needs to be modified. For example, a co-occurring disorders ACT team always had an informal working relationship with the staff of the local Section Eight housing authority. This informal relationship allowed the ACT team's staff ready access to information about waiting lists, housing availability, and any planned administrative changes. However, the Section Eight unit was moved into a new division that was hierarchical, procedurally driven, and discouraged informal communication. The ACT team's staff found that they no longer had easy and quick access to housing information. Initially this was very frustrating for both staffs who still attempted to communicate in the old manner, which resulted in several reprimands for the Section Eight unit's staff, and ACT clients ended up lower on the waiting list because proper procedures were not followed.

To counter these problems, the director of the agency of which the ACT Team is a program met with the director of the division to which the Section Eight unit belonged to develop new communication procedures between these two programs. They worked out a solution whereby the division director of the Section Eight unit gave the head of the ACT team permission to communicate directly with the head of the Section Eight unit. This is much more formal than before, but direct communications are reestablished that fall within the comfort level of the Section Eight unit's new division director.

Normally, multiple power bases exist in multilevel/multi-organization systems as follows: whoever controls the funds; whoever holds the ability to authorize the legal right for a program to provide the services; whoever has the best treatment outcomes; whoever has strong support from the political, advocacy, and professional groups in the community; and charismatic individuals who can motivate people, articulate system issues clearly, and have the respect of others. All agencies must have some power base or the support of a power base if they are to survive. When power bases in multilevel/multi-organization systems are in agreement or are willing to compromise, the system can place its total energies into the pursuit of providing effective treatment services for individuals with co-occurring disorders. However, when power bases are in disagreement and are unwilling to compromise, then energy and resources are diverted to gaining an upper hand in a power struggle.

For example, when a licensing agency and a charismatic program director, who has support from several political and advocacy power bases, engage in conflict over certain provisions of a new set of regulations, all members of the system spend a great deal of time promoting their side of the argument. The participants view this as an attempt to improve co-occurring disorders treatment services, but ego is usually the driving force and the actions taken will reduce the actual amount of time spent focusing specifically on the treatment needs of this population. On the other hand, if these different power bases are willing to make compromises about the regulations, then minimal amounts of time will be diverted from the primary functions of these organizations.

Finally, as with all human organizations, multilevel/multi-organization systems are resistant to any substantial change. Change creates uncertainty and thus discomfort for those involved, even if the change is beneficial. When substantial changes are made in a system, a period of time must be allowed for all members to express fears about this change, to accept the change, and to adapt to it.

For example, new outpatient co-occurring disorders treatment services are proposed for an existing array of services that includes existing outpatient services. The purpose of the new services is to expand the treatment system's total capacity for outpatient treatment. No jobs will be lost, no money will be shifted from other services to pay for these new ones, and more clients will have treatment services available to them. However, because a new program will provide these services a great deal of anxiety arises within the existing multilevel/multi-organization system. Questions are asked regarding why a new agency should be added to the system; referral agencies and advocate groups question the ability of the new program to provide adequate services; funding and oversight agencies wonder if they have the staff to fulfill their monitoring functions; and all wonder what it will be like working with this new program. Organizations in this system must first accept that this new program will become part of the system and that each of these questions will require time to be answered. Systems do change, but not first without a fight, and time is needed to incorporate any substantial change into the day-to-day activities of the system.

RELATIONSHIP HIERARCHIES

Normally three levels of relationships are found in multilevel/multi-organization systems. These relationships are based on hierarchical reporting arrangements. Treatment program personnel will normally report to other organizations in the system, will occasionally receive reports from other organizations, and will usually have numerous collegial reporting arrangements. How the program personnel for co-occurring disorders treatment services deal with these hierarchical relationships will greatly affect how well their program functions within this system.

Relationships with Oversight Organizations

Such relationships are usually based on contractual agreements or monitoring activities required by law. In contractual agreements, the co-occurring disorders treatment program stipulates provision of specific services for another organization, usually for some set amount of funding. Monitoring activities are typically done by federal, state, or local organizations that were established to ensure that treatment and administrative activities are conducted according to specific rules. In many ways the treatment program in this type of relationship is in a one-down position. For example, treatment program administrators may need to demonstrate to a state funding agency that a program has provided a specific number of treatment services to a specific number of clients during a specific time in order to receive full funding for services. In another instance, it may be necessary to demonstrate to a state's human rights agency that staff is fully trained concerning human rights laws and rules. In still another instance it may be necessary to demonstrate to the locally appointed advisory board that services follow best practices. How treatment program personnel handle this one-down position will affect funding, image among important power bases in the community, and legal authority to provide such services.

Such relationships can be effective or ineffective. An example of an effective one-down relationship is that of a private co-occurring disorders treatment program in which the residential treatment program had violated several state licensing requirements. The bedroom was ten square feet too small to be authorized to hold two individuals and their kitchen had several appliances that did not meet state regulations. The state inspector came down heavily by threatening to close the program. The program had only been in existence for six months and its parent agency had not run a residential program in the past. The program's management was offended by the state inspector's attitude and instinctively wanted to challenge his findings; however, they decided to approach the situation in a different manner.

The management requested a meeting with the state agency's inspector and his supervisor. The purpose of this meeting was not to challenge the findings but to acknowledge that the agency was very new to providing this type of service and to request help from the state agency in correcting these problems and preventing other problems in the future. In essence, this stand communicated that the agency wanted to work together as a team with the state agency to ensure that clients were living in an appropriate and safe environment. By taking such a stand, the program managers acknowledged the one-down position but also allowed the state agency to become an ally instead of an adversary. They tapped into the state agency's vast knowledge of how such problems had been dealt with successfully by others, how regulations might be interrupted, how other program managers found the resources to correct these problems, and found a willingness on the state agency's part to allow the program managers sufficient time to correct the problems without reducing current treatment services. Taking such stands ultimately provides better services for clients and allows program accessibility to the established system's knowledge.

Sometimes the one-down position proves ineffective. A public substance abuse treatment program provided treatment services to individuals both with and without co-occurring disorders. The program had an advisory board appointed by the local governmental body but final decisions concerning program activities were made by the director of the substance abuse program's division. The advisory board was viewed as a nuisance by both the program and division directors. They had to solicit input from the board and listen to its concerns but did not feel obliged to act on this information. This created a great deal of resentment among board members and great tension when the board meetings were held. Furthermore, influential community citizens declined appointment to the board because of its lack of power. When financial difficulties arose in the community, even if the board's membership were willing to advocate strongly against the cuts, it was usually not politically strong enough to be effective. By not acknowledging this limited, one-down position the program lost important allies in the constant struggle to maintain or expand existing funding levels.

Relationships with Organizations Receiving Oversight

Such relationships are normally contractual ones and involve an expectation that another organization will provide a specific service for clients for a set amount of funding or some other form of reimbursement. Such services may range from early prevention to long-term supportive housing. An organization manager has decided not to provide these specific services, but instead has contracted them out to another program. However, these services are ones that would be considered within this agency's responsibility to provide. For example, if the mission is to treat co-occurring disorders, then the organization managers might decide to provide outpatient treatment services but contract with another program to provide the residential portion of this treatment. The primary role of this relationship for the agency is to monitor the effectiveness of these contracted services, ensure that the allocated funds are being used appropriately, and change vendors if necessary. In this type of relationship the agency is in a one-up position. How that position is handled will greatly impact the effectiveness of the contracted services and influence the agency's ability to contract for additional services in this system in the future.

An example of an effective one-up relationship is a public behavioral health care agency that provides traditional mental health and substance abuse services and co-occurring disorders treatment, but contracts with a private agency to provide detoxification, short-term residential treatment, and transitional housing for individuals with significant substance abuse symptoms. It is expected that the contract agency will provide these services to individuals with and without co-occurring disorders. Because few organizations in the community can provide such services, only two proposals are received for this funding. Neither organization that is bidding for this service has extensive experience in providing such services. Also, since cost savings was a significant factor in deciding to outsource this service, the salaries of the staff providing these new services will be so low that the organization managers will have difficulty finding qualified people to hire. It is unlikely that these new services will be able to be effective without significant support from the public mental health and substance abuse program.

It is decided that in addition to administrative oversight of the program, a clinical supervisor with experience in these service areas will also provide oversight activities. Even though the public mental health and substance abuse program argued against outsourcing these services, they now accepted this as a reality and decided to do everything possible to make them work. Furthermore, the limited number and quality of other vendors of such services in the community made it highly unlikely that another contracted agency would do any better job. It was decided that the oversight activities would take the form of technical assistance more than the form of strict monitoring. Oversight of the administrative and clinical supervision activities of the program are done formally on a weekly basis and informal questions and discussions are encouraged on an as-needed basis. The oversight agency decides to philosophically view issues that arise during the day-to-day running of these services as ones for which the contract agency staff needs training or consultation, not punitive actions. The monitoring agency also develops jointly with the contract agency realistic and clearly measurable performance and outcome measures for the new services that demonstrate the program's progress and effectiveness. In essence, the monitoring agency views these services as an extension of their own program and takes on the ultimate responsibility for making them work. By doing so they allocated the resources necessary to support the contracted agency's development of these new services.

Example of an Ineffective One-Up Relationship

A public mental health agency contracts with a private agency to conduct its home-based case management services for individuals with and without co-occurring disorders. The contracted agency has a long relationship with the public mental health agency because it has provided group homes for mental health clients for many years on a contractual basis. The mental health agency has always been satisfied with the services that its clients received in these group homes and little monitoring of the contracted services occurred. In fact, the individual who monitors the group home contract is also a clinical supervisor and has some limited clinical responsibilities that leave very little time for contract monitoring. It is decided that this same individual will also monitor the home-based case management contract. The contract agency, unfamiliar with dealing with individuals with substance use disorders, actually helps perpetuate continued use through inappropriate case management interventions that ultimately result in the clients experiencing a crisis or losing their housing. Since little monitoring of these new services is available, the problem of a significant number of clients becoming homeless or utilizing crisis services is not detected until long after the implementation of the new contract services. An oversight agency must fulfill its monitoring function if effective treatment services are to be ensured.

Relationships with Collegial Agencies

Relationships with collegial agencies are usually based on either formal written agreements called memorandums of understanding (MOU), or informal agreements that have evolved over the years and have become more of a tradition than a formal agreement. Programs that work with individuals with co-occurring disorders receive referrals from many organizations in the community, and the program normally refers clients to other organizations that provide essential support services in the areas of social support, housing, financial, health, and employment needs. The main difference between this type of relationship and the two previously discussed is that the activities provided by independent organizations are not the program's responsibility. In these types of equal relationships interdependence exists between the treatment program and its referral sources and the treatment program and the agencies providing essential support services. How these relationships are handled will greatly affect the number of referrals and availability of support services.

Example of an Effective Collegial Relationships

An example of an effective collegial relationship involves a program providing outpatient co-occurring disorders treatment and a probation and parole office of the local district court. The district court processes less serious criminal cases including such offenses as being drunk in public, driving while intoxicated, trespassing, or disturbing the peace. The court comes into contact with many individuals who are charged for these crimes when the symptoms of their substance use or mental disorder are acute. The two programs have developed a very clear MOU that outlines who should be referred for treatment to this program, which treatment services will be provided, which reporting requirement both programs must follow, and which procedures would ensue if any of these agreements were not followed. A three-way contract (signed by the client, the therapist, and the probation officer) is developed for each referred client that outlines specific treatment services offered, client expectations, and consequences if the client did not participate appropriately in treatment. Because the procedures are clearly spelled out and are agreed to by both organizations, they are more easily followed because they are considered to be within the normal practices of these organizations. When a procedure is not followed, a clear course of action can be taken to resolve the problem. This prevents unreasonable expectations of an organization's role. It places the responsibility on the staff member to raise any issues of compliance, thus reducing the risk of simmering resentments. All these actions increase the chances that clients with criminal offenses will be provided the appropriate treatment.

Example of an Ineffective Collegial Relationship

An example of an ineffective collegial relationship involves an outpatient mental health treatment program that is structured to treat individuals with serious mental health symptoms and both serious and less serious substance use symptoms (Subgroups II and IV) and an agency that provides supportive employment services for individuals with serious mental disorders. The mental health treatment program management firmly believes that employment or volunteer work is an essential component in dealing effectively with a mental illness. Thus this program desires to refer clients to the supportive employment program as early as possible in treatment, regardless of the client's motivation toward working or volunteering and level of psychiatric stability. The supportive employment program has only a limited number of actual work slots available, staff feel very overworked, and they usually prefer that a client be psychiatrically stable and highly motivated to work or volunteer prior to being referred for services. These programs express very different views on when employment services should be offered, have had little discussion with each other concerning their philosophical viewpoints, and have no formal arrangements to work out interagency conflicts. The different views then surface in conflicts between the line staff of the mental health agency and the workers of the supportive employment agency with complaints being taken to individual supervisors but never being resolved. These issues result in many mental health therapists not referring clients regardless of their psychiatric stability or motivation for employment, or clients from the mental health agency not being accepted into the supportive employment services or being placed on very long waiting lists. Both agencies begin to be viewed in the system as not being effective in promoting employment or volunteer activities among the clients they are to serve; questions arise concerning their ability to provide these services; and clients fail to receive needed services.

CONCLUSION

This chapter focused on how almost all programs providing co-occurring disorders treatment operate in a much larger multilevel/multiorganization system that goes well beyond the traditional boundaries of mental health and substance abuse treatment systems. The chapter also discussed common characteristics found in all such systems and presented examples of these characteristics. Three types of hierarchical relationships found in these systems were also discussed and examples of effective and ineffective relationships were presented. The next chapter discusses issues that must be adequately addressed to ensure survival of programs that provide co-occurring disorders treatment services.

Chapter 10

Ensuring Service Survival

After co-occurring treatment services are established, a portion of a treatment program's time and energy must be devoted to the survival of these services, which depends on a variety of factors: funding, sufficient referrals, demonstrated treatment and cost-effectiveness, and community support. The purpose of this chapter is to explore each of these aspects that contribute to program survival and make recommendations concerning how they can be most effectively achieved.

ENSURING ADEQUATE AND ONGOING FUNDING

Without funding, programs for co-occurring disorders treatment services cannot exist. The more diversified the funding sources, the greater the survivability of treatment services. Services based on single funding sources are always vulnerable to termination should the funding source cease to exist or choose to invest its money on different priorities. Currently the vast majority of funding for co-occurring disorders treatment services comes from federal, state, or local monies designated for mental health and substance abuse treatment services. However, health insurance, private endowments, and client fees may also play an important part in program revenue. Although funding sources are limited, one goal of any program that provides treatment services to this population should be to diversify its funding sources as much as possible.

Funding Diversification

Funding diversification can be achieved in three ways. The first method of diversification involves reallocating existing funds designated for a specific activity related to co-occurring disorders treatment but not specifically marked for that type of treatment. For example, portions of monies received for substance abuse or mental health treatment from the Federal State Block Grant Program could be reallocated to provide treatment services for individuals with co-occurring disorders. Any such reallocation must meet legal, ethical, and statements of intent if they are to serve the program well in the long run. In this case the federal government has declared that these funds can be used to treat individuals with co-occurring disorders (Substance Abuse and Mental Health Services Administration's Report to Congress, 2002), thus any reallocation would meet legal requirements. Ethically the program can justify that the portion of money being reallocated will continue to provide the service for which it was originally intended, because mental health or substance abuse treatment services will continue to be provided to these clients. However, a portion of it will be used immediately to provide co-occurring disorders treatment services to those clients who need such services. Thus the portion of money being reallocated would only reflect the actual percentage of existing clients in need of this service. Such an action does not take money away for clients in need, but in fact provides the actual services that clients truly need. The third part of this process involves announcing the intention to use these funds for co-occurring disorders treatment services along with the justifications for doing so to the necessary authorities prior to taking the action. In this case, the necessary authority would usually be the state, which administers these funds. This allows the funding authorities the opportunity for buy in or at least advanced warning so such activities would not come to their attention in an embarrassing manner.

The reallocation process discussed here can theoretically be done with any existing funding source for mental health and substance abuse treatment funds. All programs providing substance abuse and mental health treatment have clients with co-occurring disorders. Reallocating existing funds to treat these co-occurring disorders conditions is simply acknowledging the realities of the current treatment environment. Obviously the legal use of such funds will be different depending on the funding source; however, it is imperative that program managers find out about the legality of using funds from all their funding sources for providing co-occurring disorders treatment services, and when it is illegal to lobby for a change in that legal status. The statements of intent must always be presented in a collaborative manner. Combative statements can only serve to entrench the funding authority into a "no position." The goal of this part of the process is that at worst the program and its funding authority respectfully agree to disagree. By tapping into existing funding sources, no new monies are needed to provide the treatment services that a percentage of any program's existing clients need, and an existing funding source for this population is solidified.

The second method of funding diversification involves identifying new or expanding existing sources of revenue. For example, federal and state agencies normally target some portion of their budgets to fund special projects. The special project funds are usually time limited and targeted to new services. These funds offer programs the opportunity to establish new services for individuals with co-occurring disorders. Because these funds are limited, program administrators must be able to demonstrate that they can use them effectively. Usually very little time elapses between the announcement that the funds are available and the deadline for application. Few programs have the resources to respond rapidly to the requests for proposals (RFPs), so a plan must be in place for responding to these announcements prior to their posting. Most RFPs have similar formats and require similar information. This includes program description and history of providing treatment services, proposed services, staffing patterns, budgets and the ability to manage them, methods for evaluating effectiveness of new services, and letters of community support. Much of this information can be compiled in a working format ahead of time, so that responding to an RFP can be done in a manner that does not require the program to significantly reduce the time it dedicates to other activities. Approaching RFPs in such a manner allows even small programs to solicit additional funding through the RFP process.

The third method of funding diversification involves the creative use of monies that fund support services frequently used by this population. This money may be used to expand services or to make these services more specific to the needs of individuals with co-occurring disorders. As in the case of reallocation, creative use of these funds must be done legally, ethically, and with an honest statement of intention to the funding source. For example, some of the funds that an agency receives for the homeless might be used to establish a group home for homeless individuals with co-occurring disorders. Since this population has high homelessness rates, the funding source expresses no difficulty using the money for this purpose. Residents of the new group home are connected with the agency's outpatient co-occurring disorders treatment services and the group home counselors receive special training for working with this population. Using monies allocated for services allows the agency to expand its continuum of care for individuals with co-occurring disorders.

In another instance, some money used to fund services for welfare-to-work participants is used to hire an on-site therapist to provide substance abuse, mental health, and co-occurring disorders treatment. The case is made with the state social service department that significant numbers of their participants in this service have these disorders and if the disorders are not successfully treated it is unlikely they will be successful participants in these other services. In addition, the case is made that these treatment services would be most utilized if they were offered at the same site where other welfare-to-work services are provided because the local mental health and substance abuse treatment programs do not have sufficient staff to place a therapist on-site. To support these services, the local agency that normally provided co-occurring disorders treatment services to this population agrees to provide the clinical supervision for the new on-site therapist. Hence, part of the welfare-to-work funding is used to increase the treatment capacity for this population.

In still another instance, monies used to fund employment support services in a community are used to target special needs of individuals with co-occurring disorders. The employment services agency finds that it is ineffective when individuals with high psychiatric and/or substance abuse symptoms (including individuals in Subgroups II, III, and IV) use their services, and that these individuals are at times disruptive. The treatment agencies in the community who provide treatment services for this population offer to train one of the employment specialists to work effectively with these individuals and offer space in their facilities so that these individuals no longer need go to the employment agency's location. In this example, employment funds are used to increase the availability of specialized services for individuals with co-occurring disorders.

Each of these methods of funding diversification needs to be utilized if the broadest foundation of funding for co-occurring disorders treatment services is to be established. These methods use existing sources of revenue, identify potential new ones, and creatively make use of other forms of funding to help reduce dependence on single or limited sources of funding. Ensuring funding is an ongoing process that needs constant attention, and occurs in a social environment that is constantly changing its priorities and the rules that govern the use of funds for mental health, substance abuse, and other related human services. A treatment program must dedicate some of its human resources to the task of diversifying funding sources if it is to survive in the long run.

ENSURING SUFFICIENT REFERRALS

Without an adequate number of referrals a program cannot justify its existence. For a referral source to use a treatment service it must perceive that its clients are in need of such services; that these services are effective; and that they can establish and maintain a professional working relationship with the treatment program. As with the case of funding, having diversified referral sources increases the chances of adequate census levels. Traditional referral sources for co-occurring disorders treatment services include the following:

- other mental health and substance abuse treatment programs;
- the criminal justice system;
- social service agencies;
- homeless programs;
- employment services; and
- health care services.

Each co-occurring treatment program must develop working relationships with these and other potential referral sources in the community if they are to secure an adequate number of clients.

Most of the traditional referral agencies have some level of experience in identifying and referring for treatment individuals with mental health and substance use disorders. However, few will have the experience needed to determine who should receive specialized treatment for co-occurring disorders. When these services are initiated within existing mental health and substance abuse treatment programs, this diagnostic issue is resolved internally. During the admission process it can be decided if the client is to be provided co-occurring disorders treatment. However, when such services are offered through a new stand-alone program, determining who to refer where is much more complicated for referral agencies. Two steps can be taken to successfully address this referral issue.

First, the stand-alone co-occurring disorders treatment program must develop written admission criteria that provide clear descriptions of appropriate candidates for their services, with suggestions concerning how to determine if an individual has co-occurring disorders. Second, the new program should then present these criteria to existing substance abuse and mental health treatment programs prior to advertising their services to other traditional referral agencies.

Existing mental health and substance abuse treatment programs are critical partners in ensuring that clients with co-occurring disorders are referred to new stand-alone programs. These mental health and substance abuse treatment programs will continue to have individuals with co-occurring disorders referred to them; however, if they are familiar with the new program and its admission criteria they will be able to redirect referral agencies to these new services. There is usually strong motivation to do this on the part of existing treatment programs, because otherwise they are the recipients of many inappropriate referrals. This also generates referrals of existing clients in these treatment agencies who have co-occurring disorders. Once this step has been completed, the new stand-alone program can approach other referral sources and provide them with an in-depth overview of their services and admission criteria. Initially, it will be important that the new stand-alone program identify at least one staff member who can serve as liaison to existing mental health and substance abuse treatment programs and other referral sources to answer any specific questions they have concerning who should be referred to their services.

Before an agency refers a client to co-occurring disorders treatment services, it must perceive that the client will benefit from this referral. A variety of performance standards and outcome measures are used to demonstrate co-occurring disorders treatment effectiveness. These are reviewed in the next section of this chapter. As in the previous case, existing programs that initiate co-occurring disorders treatment services have already demonstrated their effectiveness to referral agencies over the years by means of actual outcome numbers or from anecdotal evidence of numerous referred cases that were successfully treated. New stand-alone co-occurring disorders treatment programs have neither outcome numbers nor a history of providing successful services for clients of these referral agencies. In this situation, the new program must use outcome numbers from research studies and demonstrate that they are using the treatment practices that generated these outcomes. The next section of this chapter reviews treatment outcome findings for this population. Chapter 2 reviewed the qualities of an effective co-occurring disorders treatment program. This information can be used to promote reasonable treatment outcome expectations for new co-occurring disorders treatment services and ensure that referred clients will receive state-of-the-art treatment.

The ongoing working relationship between the program providing the co-occurring disorders treatment services and the referral agency is ultimately the key to a steady flow of clients. This relationship is not only based on trust that clients will receive effective treatment but that the referral agency will also receive what it needs. Referral agencies always need regular reporting of their clients' participation and progress in treatment. Such reports allow them to demonstrate that they are monitoring their clients' participation in needed services and provide them with the ability to take necessary actions in a timely manner (such as returning a client to court for nonparticipation in treatment). To meet this need, co-occurring disorders treatment programs must develop a reporting system to referral agencies that adequately meets their information needs and is within the administrative capacity of the program. Reporting requirements can vary greatly from regular formal written reports, to occasional informal phone calls, to just a discharge summary at the end of treatment. The important issue is that the referral agency receive the information it needs to do its job.

Again, when new co-occurring disorders services are introduced into existing mental health and substance abuse treatment programs, reporting requirements to referral agencies and methods of resolving differences of opinion concerning clinical interventions are usually already in place. However, when a new stand-alone program is established, specific reporting requirements and methods of resolving clinical differences must be developed for each referral agency. A single meeting with staff of that agency, often at the time the new services are presented, can be used to develop reporting requirements. Clinical differences of opinion usually need to be resolved through facilitated face-to-face discussion among the relevant staff. Since reports will not always be submitted on time and periodic clinical differences will occur between referral and treatment agencies, co-occurring disorders treatment programs must establish a process for responding to these issues. These responses include the following:

- The clinical supervisors sign off on all reports to monitor their timeliness.
- Supervisors of clinical services and referral agencies maintain regular communications that include concerns about inadequate reporting.
- Supervisors and staff meet jointly to work out perceived clinical differences.
- All the staff of these programs meet periodically to address any issues that exist between them.

By establishing a process to work out clinical differences, submitting process reports on time, demonstrating treatment effectiveness, and helping referral agencies to identify clients in need of services, co-occurring disorders treatment programs will ensure an adequate client base.

DEMONSTRATING COST
AND TREATMENT EFFECTIVENESS

Sources of funding, referral, and political support need proof that their funds, their clients, or their energy are being wisely spent and that persons in need are receiving effective treatment services. The primary manner in which programs provide this proof is to compare their projected performance and outcome numbers to the actual numbers achieved. Performance measures examine the number of clients served, number of services provided, days in treatment, etc. Outcome measures include percentage of clients engaged in treatment, percentage of clients completing treatment, percentage of clients with no additional contact with the criminal justice system, and so forth. The purpose of this section is to examine the substantial research that documents the effectiveness of substance abuse, mental health, and co-occurring disorders treatment; review common performance and outcome measures used to document this effectiveness; explain how current measures came into use; and provide benchmarks for programs to use to develop reasonable performance and treatment outcome expectations.

Substance Abuse, Mental Health, and Co-Occurring Disorders Treatment Outcome Studies

Research concerning co-occurring disorders treatment outcomes has evolved from traditional studies of substance abuse and mental health treatment outcomes. The federal government has sponsored five major national studies concerning the effectiveness of substance abuse treatment in public programs (Gerstein et al., 1994; Hubbard et al., 1989; Hubbard et al., 1997; Substance Abuse and Mental Health Services Administration, 1994; Simpson and Sells, 1982). Another major study examined the effectiveness of private substance abuse treatment programs (Hoffman and Miller, 1992) and twenty-four states have conducted major studies on the effectiveness of their substance abuse treatment services (Gerstein et al., 1994; National Association of State Alcohol and Drug Abuse Directors, 2002). The United Kingdom also has conducted a major study of the effectiveness of that nation's substance abuse treatment programs (Gossop et al., 1997). Each study found that substance abuse treatment provides many benefits to both the individual and society, all of which can be used as outcome measures. The following list summarizes these findings:

- Reduced drug use
- Reduced criminal activities
- Reduced health costs
- Reduced homelessness
- Reduced suicide attempts
- Reduced food stamp needs
- Reduced child welfare cases
- Increased employment and earnings

The scope of mental health issues that receives treatment attention (from major mental disorders, such as schizophrenia, to personal growth) and the many variations in treatment approaches make it impossible to conduct large national studies of multiple treatment programs, as has been done in the substance abuse field. Whereas substance abuse programs deal with either abuse or dependence, disorders, and generally have treatment goals of either abstinence or nonproblematic substance use, mental health treatment programs address multiple conditions that have many differing treatment goals. Thus, mental health outcome research focuses on specific conditions that have specific treatment goals. As with substance abuse research studies, mental health treatment studies have found that medication, behavioral, and talk therapies all are effective in improving both the daily functioning and the quality of life for individuals with these disorders (U.S. Public Health Service, 2001). This is particularly true when they are used in combination.

Although outcome studies of individuals receiving treatment for co-occurring disorders have not been as extensive as for individuals who have received traditional mental health and substance abuse treatment services, the results have been similar. Outcome studies concerning this population have examined outpatient services (Bond et al., 1991; Drake, McHugo, and Noordsy, 1993; Hellerstein, Rosenthal, and Miner, 1995); intensive or assertive community treatment services (Drake et al., 1998; Durell et al., 1993; Meisler et al., 1997); and residential treatment services (Bartels and Drake, 1996; Mierlak et al., 1998). These studies find that treatment, when modified to meet the special needs of individuals with co-occurring disorders, also provide many benefits for these clients and society. The following list summarizes these findings and provides potential outcome measures for the treatment of co-occurring disorders.

- Reduced substance use
- Reduced psychiatric symptoms
- Reduced hospitalizations
- Increased use of appropriate treatment services
- Increased stabilized housing
- Improved quality of life

Measuring Changes in Substance Use and Mental Health Symptoms

Client change during treatment and maintaining that change is a measure often used to demonstrate program effectiveness. The three methods that I have found most helpful for measuring change among individuals with co-occurring disorders are Client Readiness for Change (Prochaska, DiClemente, and Norcoss, 1992); Substance Abuse Treatment Scale (Mueser et al., 1995); and Tracking Changes Toward Abstinence and Recovery (Hendrickson, Stith, and Schmal, 1995). The latter two were developed specifically for individuals with co-occurring disorders. Each measures different aspects of client change and requires only a minimum amount of time and resources to document. A description of each and the client changes they identify are as follows.

Client Readiness for Change

This five-stage model measures clients' readiness for behavior change. These stages are labeled precontemplation, contemplation, preparation, action, and maintenance. Precontemplation indicates that the client has neither interest in treatment nor any intention to change behavior. In the contemplation stage, the client is aware of a problem and thinks he or she might want to overcome it in the future. Preparation is the stage in which the client intends to take action and begins to plan how to do that. In the action stage, the client is in treatment and modifying behavior. Maintenance is the stage during which the client works to prevent relapse and consolidate gains. This client readiness for change can be easily measured through the publicly available thirty-two-item questionnaire, Change Assessment Scale, which can be administered and scored in a short time. This measure allows mental health and substance abuse therapists to track changes in clients' acceptance of a problem and their willingness to make or maintain behavioral changes.

Substance Abuse Treatment Scale

This eight-stage model is based on a four-stage model originally proposed by Osher and Kofoed (1989) and measures clients' level of participation in treatment and decreases in substance use. This model divides each of Osher and Kofoed's four stages of engagement, persuasion, active treatment, and relapse prevention into early or late stages. During the pre-engagement stage, the potential client has no contact with a treatment professional. During the engagement stage, the client has irregular contact with a treatment professional. In the early persuasion stage, the client has regular contact with a treatment professional but has not changed the substance use. The late persuasion stage involves regular contact with a treatment professional and clients' discussing their substance use and reducing use somewhat. The early active treatment stage involves, in addition to the activities noted in the late persuasion stage, a stated goal of working toward abstinence. The late active treatment stage occurs when the client has achieved abstinence for less than six months. In the relapse prevention stage, abstinence has been achieved for six months. Occasional lapses are allowed in this stage but not days of relapse or problematic use. The final stage, remission or recovery, is achieved when the client has had no substance use problems for over a year and is no longer in treatment for the substance use disorder. This model allows therapists to measure changes in both treatment participation and substance use behavior.

Tracking Changes Toward Abstinence and Recovery

This model measures observable changes in clients' behavior and expressions of attitudes and motivation concerning substance use. Each of its five stages is a specific substance use behavior, attitude, and motivation toward substance use. In the first stage, substance use behaviors continue with no acknowledgment that substance use is a problem and the client has no motivation to abstain. In the second stage, a client abstains as a result of outside pressure (such as the court or family), but does not acknowledge that use is a problem and has no motivation to abstain if the outside pressure is discontinued. In the third stage, a client acknowledges that use is a problem but the use continues and there is no motivation expressed for abstinence. In the fourth stage, the substance use continues but the client acknowledges that use is a problem and expresses a desire to achieve abstinence. The fifth and final stage is reached when the client achieves abstinence, acknowledges that use is a problem, and expresses a desire to continue abstinence. This model allows therapists to track changes in clients during the normal course of treatment.

Each of these models provides therapists and treatment agencies with methods to measure change during a specific treatment episode and to provide a basis for determining positive treatment outcomes from negative treatment outcomes. Treatment agencies or professionals must determine how to classify a treatment success. Is any positive movement from one stage to another during treatment considered a successful treatment event, or must a specific amount of positive change take place before treatment is considered successful? One treatment professional or agency might decide that only abstinence should be considered a treatment success; another might see the reduction of substance use or moving from denial to accepting that substance use is a problem as success; still others might see moving from refusing treatment to accepting treatment services as a treatment success. Of course, these are philosophical questions, but they need to be answered before treatment outcomes can be measured. Obviously, the higher the standards, the lower the success rates will be, which is an important factor for individual therapists and agencies to consider when establishing performance standards.

Predicting Treatment Outcome

As discussed earlier in this chapter, treatment for substance use and mental disorders has been found to be overwhelmingly more effective than no treatment. A variety of factors contributes to positive treatment outcomes. Research finds seven variables linked to positive treatment outcomes for substance abuse treatment: longer treatment stays, being older, being employed, being married, family involvement in treatment, participation in self-help groups and, for narcotic addicts, having the proper methadone dosage (Ball and Ross, 1991; Hartell et al., 1995; Hoffman, Harrison, and Belille, 1983; Hubbard et al., 1989; Mammo and Weinbaum, 1993; McCrady et al., 1986; O'Farrel, 1989; Ornstein and Cherepon, 1985; Simpson and Sells, 1982; Vallant, 1983; Westermeyer, 1989). Similar factors have been found to contribute to positive treatment outcomes for individuals with co-occurring mental disorders (Bond et al., 1991; Hendrickson, Stith, Schmal, 1995; Maisto et al., 1999). Factors associated with positive mental health outcomes vary from disorder to disorder. However, medication compliance is a critical one for many disorders.

Of these variables, the key predicting variable for individuals with a substance use disorder appears to be *retention in treatment,* both for individuals with and without co-occurring mental disorders. In general, the longer an individual stays in treatment the better the progress. Findings from several large substance abuse treatment outcome studies (Hubbard et al., 1989; Hubbard et al., 1997; Simpson and Sells, 1982), indicate that ninety days' retention in treatment is the critical threshold that predicts long-term substance abuse changes— both for outpatient treatment and residential treatment. The critical threshold for methadone maintenance was one-year retention. A study by Hendrickson and Schmal (2000) also indicates that ninety days' retention is the critical threshold for predicting positive treatment outcome for individuals with co-occurring serious mental illness and substance use disorders. These studies also find that as retention extends beyond ninety days, success rates continue to increase. Fortunately, individual therapists and treatment program procedures can easily measure treatment retention or completion rates with few, if any, changes in the current way they keep information about their clients. The next sections review national averages and make recommendations concerning the performance standards that individuals or agencies can use to measure their treatment effectiveness.

Retention Rates

The major national substance abuse studies (Hubbard et al., 1989; Hubbard et al., 1997; Simpson and Sells, 1982) find that 36 to 57 percent of individuals in outpatient treatment stay in treatment ninety days or more; 42 to 53 percent of individuals in long-term residential treatment stay in treatment ninety days or more; and 34 to 50 percent of individuals stay in methadone maintenance for one year or more.

Client retention in treatment programs for individuals with co-occurring disorders were similar. The range for ninety days' retention in outpatient treatment was 34 to 47 percent (Bennett, Bellack, and Gearson, 2000; Case, 1991; Drake, McHugo, and Noordsy, 1993; Hanson, Kramer and Gross, 1990; Hendrickson and Schmal, 2000; Kofoed et al., 1986); the retention in residential treatment, although only reported at six months, ranged from 34 to 37 percent (Bartels and Drake, 1996; Mierlak et al., 1998). Thus we can speculate that ninety-day rates would be similar because most residential treatment dropouts occur within the first thirty days. Information concerning retention on methadone maintenance by individuals with co-occurring disorders has not been reported.

Readmission Rates

Although readmission rates are often viewed as a negative treatment outcome, several substance abuse studies (Hubbard et al., 1989; Simpson and Sells, 1982) indicate that accumulative treatment time can be as effective as a single treatment episode. Thus readmission can ultimately contribute to a positive treatment outcome. So what might individual therapists and treatment programs expect concerning the readmission rates of their clients?

All but the initial national substance abuse studies find that 54 to 59 percent of clients entering substance abuse treatment had been in some form of substance abuse treatment prior to that admission. Because the Drug Abuse Reporting Program (DARP) study covered the period (1969-1973) when treatment programs for substance abuse were just developing and when most users of drugs other than alcohol had recently begun their use, it can be assumed that its lower readmission figure (40 percent) was more the result of the lack of long-term drug use and the scarcity of treatment resources. Treatment Episode Data (TED) (Substance Abuse Mental Health Services Administration, 1998), which maintains information on substance abuse treatment programs receiving federal funding, reports that the more intensive the treatment service, the more likely that it is not the client's first admission. Thirty percent of clients admitted to outpatient programs had prior substance abuse treatment services, while 50 percent of clients admitted to residential programs, and 70 percent of individuals admitted to methadone programs had prior treatment admissions.

Readmission rates for individuals with co-occurring disorders are not well studied. A study by Hendrickson and Schmal (2000), which explored readmission rates of this population to outpatient treatment groups over an eighteen-year period, showed that the average length of time between the first and second group treatment admission was approximately thirty-two months and 95 percent of the second admissions occurred within 7.5 years. Using that 7.5 year time frame as a benchmark, they estimate the readmission rate to these groups to be 41 percent. This did not include admissions to other treatment programs. Thus the true readmission rate for this population is higher and possibly similar to the readmission rates for general substance abuse treatment programs. Client change, retention, and readmission studies offer important benchmarks that can help treatment professionals and programs determine if they are performing as well as other professionals and programs across the nation.

Reasonable Performance Standards

Performance standards allow therapists or treatment programs to compare what they desire to achieve with their actual performance. Performance standards should always be based on research concerning national averages, the nature of the treatment population, and the resources available to the agency or therapist. Programs that have lower client/staff ratios, a fully funded continuum of care, and a client population that is generally compliant with treatment would be expected to set higher performance standards than the national average, while programs with limited resources and a very resistant and noncompliant treatment population might establish lower performance standards than the national average. The three most important performance standards that all therapists and programs working with individuals with co-occurring disorders can easily measure are the rates of retention, readmission, and client change during treatment.

ESTABLISHING AND MAINTAINING COMMUNITY SUPPORT

Community support involves establishing and maintaining effective relationships with the political, advocacy, and professional groups that operate within the jurisdictions served by the program's co-occurring disorders treatment services. Without this support the program will not be able to survive funding cuts, changes in community priorities, or clinical mistakes. Political groups normally advocate how local taxes will be used by elected officials of local government bodies such as city councils, county, or township boards. Advocacy groups promote sufficient and quality mental health and substance abuse treatment services or community awareness of the consequences of these disorders and include organizations such as local alliances for the mentally ill, local advocates for substance abuse treatment, or Mothers Against Drunk Driving (MADD). Professional groups represent the interests of the staff providing the treatment services and include local branches of such organizations as the National Association of Social Workers (NASW), National Association of Alcohol and Drug Abuse Counselors (NADAC), or the American Psychological Association (APA). Each program must develop a strategy for interacting effectively with each of these groups if the program is to receive professional group support.

The first step of any effective strategy for gaining support from these groups is to understand what interest and positions the group represents. The program can then interact with the groups in a thoughtful and constructive manner. Interactions with these community groups result from information requests about the program's services or as a response to some criticism of the program.

For example, the local city council, which funds 30 percent of new co-occurring disorders treatment services, requests information outside the normal budget process concerning client usage of these services. The program management is aware that the city is considering budget cuts to avoid raising taxes, so they rightly assume that some portion of their funding is being considered for a cut. Their response is threefold. First, they promptly respond to the city council's request by providing performance and outcome data about their services that demonstrates usage of the services, the effectiveness of the services, and the cost benefits these services provide the community. Second, they also alert friendly advocacy and professional groups that the city council might be considering reducing or eliminating funds for their co-occurring treatment services, and provide these groups the same information that was given to the city council. These support groups now have information that they can use if lobbying is necessary. The third step is an internal process that involves reviewing the program's existing funding structure to determine if ways to continue the services at the current level are available if budget cuts are made. By documenting the effectiveness of the services, promoting lobbying efforts if necessary, and exploring alternative funding methods, the program greatly increases the chances that the services will not be reduced.

In another example, a local mental health advocacy group generated a public statement criticizing some of the treatment practices used by a program that provided co-occurring disorders treatment services. Specifically, they were critical of the practice of sharing urine test results with probation officers, that certain medications were not provided to some clients, and that some clients were terminated from treatment for refusing to address certain issues. The mental health advocacy group firmly believed that these practices violated the human dignity of these individuals and their innate right to receive the type of treatment they choose. Instead of attacking the advocacy group for misrepresenting what they do, the treatment program's management decided that this criticism was the result of their failure to communicate clearly to this group about the clinical reasons for these treatment practices. They reached out to the group and proposed a meeting. The purpose of this meeting was to listen to the reasons why the advocacy group decided to publicly take this position and to provide the program with an opportunity to explain to this group the clinical reasons behind these treatment practices.

This meeting might not result in either a change in a position or practices; however, it will increase an understanding of why each group believes as it does. It also has the potential to develop an ongoing dialogue and relationship between the two organizations, which at a minimum can create an atmosphere of respectful disagreement between them in the community. It is not necessary that advocacy groups endorse all the practices of co-occurring disorders treatment services; however, it is important that these groups understand that accepted clinical reasons lie behind these practices and that program personnel are not behaving unprofessionally.

In still another example, a client of a co-occurring disorders treatment program committed suicide after failing to receive medication for depression in a timely manner. The client's family was very angry about this, and the entire story was published in the local newspaper. As a result, the program came under intense scrutiny by local political, advocacy, and professional groups. In this instance, instead of defending the quality of their services, the program managers publicly pledged to thoroughly investigate the incident and take any needed corrective actions. To ensure public confidence in this investigation, the program administrators invited representatives from each of these groups to be part of the investigation. The case was examined thoroughly, mistakes that were made were openly acknowledged, and procedures were put in place to prevent this occurrence in the future.

Clinical mistakes will be made and the co-occurring disordered population is a very high-risk group. It is most important that these mistakes be acknowledged when they occur, that they are viewed as learning experiences, and procedures are developed for preventing them in the future. Maintaining support from local community groups involves keeping the groups informed about the program's activities; being willing to work cooperatively with them; being forthcoming about program limitations or mistakes; and making changes when needed. Doing so makes the treatment program part of a community team instead of an unknown entity or adversary.

CONCLUSION

Without sufficient funding, referrals, and community support a program providing treatment services for individuals with co-occurring disorders will cease to exist. To ensure this support, a program must demonstrate both cost and treatment effectiveness. This chapter presented a variety of ways to ensure funding diversity, sufficient referrals, adequate community support, and methods of demonstrating program effectiveness. Programs that provide services for this population have a wide range of issues to deal with on a day-to-day basis. This section provides to the direct service provider, the clinical supervisor, and the manager ideas and strategies that can make their jobs easier.

Section IV:
Appendixes

This section provides the reader with the basic tools needed to conduct comprehensive community needs assessment of co-occurring disorders treatment services; conduct effective interviews of applicants for co-occurring disorders treatment positions; and conduct training needs assessment of staff providing such services. Appendix A provides the forms necessary to identify all the existing co-occurring disorders treatment services being provided by local substance abuse, mental health, and co-occurring disorders treatment services providers. In addition, a form is included in Appendix A that summarizes all existing co-occurring disorders treatment services in the community and identifies gaps in such services. How such information can be solicited and used is discussed in detail in Chapter 3 of this book. Appendix B provides sample interview questions for applicants for co-occurring disorders treatment positions; case examples of each of the four subgroups of individuals with co-occurring disorders; and an Applicant Assessment Form that can be used to summarize the applicant's documented and observed experience, knowledge and skill levels. Appendix C provides a self-report training assessment form for staff providing treatment services to individuals with co-occurring disorders. This form measures both perceived knowledge and skill levels and training interest in all topics relevant to providing effective treatment services for this population. Chapter 6 discusses in detail the applicant hiring process and developing staff training programs. Readers should feel free to modify any of the forms in these appendixes to meet the specific needs of their program or community.

Appendix A

Model Community Needs Assessment

The purpose of this appendix is to provide the reader with a needs assessment package that can be used to help a community identify which co-occurring disorders treatment services are currently provided, as well as any gaps existing in the services. The tool is composed of four forms. The first three forms are separate needs assessment forms for each existing substance abuse, mental health, or co-occurring disorders treatment program in the community, which help identify all existing traditional and specialized co-occurring disorder services throughout the entire continuum of care. They identify specific portions of the continuum of care currently in place for individuals with and without co-occurring disorders, which specific services each program provides, which subgroups of individuals with co-occurring disorders are provided services, the program's treatment capacity, existing links with essential supportive services, qualities that a program processed, and the program administration's willingness to expand or add co-occurring disorders services. A fourth form is also included in the needs assessment package that provides one central location where all collected information can be compiled. This form offers a complete picture of all co-occurring disorders treatment services currently offered in the community, which portions of this population are receiving these services, gaps that exist in treatment capacity and the continuum of care, and if current treatment program administrators are willing to fill these gaps. Chapter 3 provides detailed information about conducting community needs assessments that can be used in planning for co-occurring disorders treatment services.

NEEDS ASSESSMENT FORM: SUBSTANCE ABUSE PROGRAM

SUBSTANCE ABUSE PROGRAM:

Location: _____ (Adm Req) **Age** _____ **Gender** _____ **Residency** _____

CURRENT CONTINUUM OF CARE COMPONENTS OFFERED

Components	C/O/D Served/Type[a]	Services[b] Ind Gp CM Fam Med	#FTEs/Static/Annual[c]	Community Links[d] H F M E
Pretreatment				
Prevention	No / Yes I, II, III, IV	— — — — —	/ / / /	— — — —
Outreach	No / Yes I, II, III, IV	— — — — —	/ / / /	— — — —
Early Intervention	No / Yes I, II, III, IV	— — — — —	/ / / /	— — — —
Outpatient				
Intensive Day	No / Yes I, II, III, IV	— — — — —	/ / / /	— — — —
Intensive Tx	No / Yes I, II, III, IV	— — — — —	/ / / /	— — — —
Outpatient Tx	No / Yes I, II, III, IV	— — — — —	/ / / /	— — — —
Opiate Replacement	No / Yes I, II, III, IV	— — — — —	/ / / /	— — — —
Residential/Inpatient				
Medical Detox	No / Yes I, II, III, IV	— — — — —	/ / / /	— — — —
Nonmedical Detox	No / Yes I, II, III, IV	— — — — —	/ / / /	— — — —
Residential (−90 days)	No / Yes I, II, III, IV	— — — — —	/ / / /	— — — —
Residential (90+ days)	No / Yes I, II, III, IV	— — — — —	/ / / /	— — — —
Supportive Housing	No / Yes I, II, III, IV	— — — — —	/ / / /	— — — —
Other _____	No / Yes I, II, III, IV	— — — — —	/ / /	— — — —
Other _____	No / Yes I, II, III, IV	— — — — —	/ / /	— — — —

ADDITIONAL INFORMATION ON _____ (Program's Name)

Observed Qualities

Accessibility of Services	Yes No	Comments:
Integrated Treatment	Yes No	Comments:
Competency-Based View	Yes No	Comments:
Treatment Flexibility	Yes No	Comments:
Variable Stays	Yes No	Comments:

Willingness to Add/Expand and Co-Occurring Tx Services: Yes No

What Types of Services: _____

What Is Needed to Add/Expand the Services: _____

_____

_____

Additional Comments:

[a]C/O/D – co-occurring disorder

[b]Ind – Individual; Gp = Group; CM = _____ ; Fam = Family; Med = Medical

[c]FTE = full-time equivalents

[d]H = housing; F = financial; M = medical; E = employment

NEEDS ASSESSMENT FORM: MENTAL HEALTH PROGRAM

MENTAL HEALTH PROGRAM:

Location: _____ (Adm Req) Age _____ Gender _____ Residency _____

CURRENT CONTINUUM OF CARE COMPONENTS OFFERED

Components	C/O/D Served/Type[a]	Services[b] Ind Gp CM Fam Med	#FTEs/Static /Annual[c]	Community Links[d] H F M E
Pretreatment				
Prevention	No / Yes I, II, III, IV	__ __ __ __ __	/ /	__ __ __ __
Outreach	No / Yes I, II, III, IV	__ __ __ __ __	/ /	__ __ __ __
Early Intervention	No / Yes I, II, III, IV	__ __ __ __ __	/ /	__ __ __ __
Outpatient				
Intensive Day	No / Yes I, II, III, IV	__ __ __ __ __	/ /	__ __ __ __
Intensive Tx	No / Yes I, II, III, IV	__ __ __ __ __	/ /	__ __ __ __
Outpatient Tx	No / Yes I, II, III, IV	__ __ __ __ __	/ /	__ __ __ __
Psychosocial	No / Yes I, II, III, IV	__ __ __ __ __	/ /	__ __ __ __
ACT Team	No / Yes I, II, III, IV	__ __ __ __ __	/ /	__ __ __ __
Medication Only	No / Yes I, II, III, IV	__ __ __ __ __	/ /	__ __ __ __
Residential/Inpatient				
Crisis Intervention	No / Yes I, II, III, IV	__ __ __ __ __	/ /	__ __ __ __
Crisis Stabilization	No / Yes I, II, III, IV	__ __ __ __ __	/ /	__ __ __ __
Hospitalization	No / Yes I, II, III, IV	__ __ __ __ __	/ /	__ __ __ __
Supportive Housing	No / Yes I, II, III, IV	__ __ __ __ __	/ /	__ __ __ __
Other _____	No / Yes I, II, III, IV	__ __ __ __ __	/ /	__ __ __ __
Other _____	No / Yes I, II, III, IV	__ __ __ __ __	/ /	__ __ __ __

ADDITIONAL INFORMATION ON _____ (Program's Name)

Observed Qualities

Accessibility   Yes No   Comments:
of Services

Integrated   Yes No   Comments:
   Treatment

Competency   Yes No   Comments:
Based View

Treatment   Yes No   Comments:
Flexibility

Variable   Yes No   Comments:
Stays

Willingness to Add/Expand and Co-Occurring Tx Services: Yes   No

What Types of Services: _____

What Is Needed to Add/Expand the Services: _____

_____

_____

Additional Comments:

[a]C/O/D – co-occurring disorder

[b]Ind – Individual; Gp = Group; CM = _____ ; Fam = Family; Med = Medical

[c]FTE = full-time equivalents

[d]H = housing; F = financial; M = medical; E = employment

NEEDS ASSESSMENT FORM: CO-OCCURRING DISORDERS PROGRAM

CO-OCCURRING DISORDERS PROGRAM:

Location: _____ (Adm Req) Age _____ Gender _____ Residency _____

CURRENT CONTINUUM OF CARE COMPONENTS OFFERED

Components	C/O/D Type[a]	Services[b] (Ind Gp CM Fam Med)	#FTEs/Static/Annual[c]	Community Links[d] (H F M E)
Pretreatment				
Prevention	I, II, III, IV	___ ___ ___ ___ ___	/ /	___ ___ ___ ___
Outreach	I, II, III, IV	___ ___ ___ ___ ___	/ /	___ ___ ___ ___
Early Intervention	I, II, III, IV	___ ___ ___ ___ ___	/ /	___ ___ ___ ___
Outpatient				
Intensive Day	I, II, III, IV	___ ___ ___ ___ ___	/ /	___ ___ ___ ___
Intensive Tx	I, II, III, IV	___ ___ ___ ___ ___	/ /	___ ___ ___ ___
Outpatient Tx	I, II, III, IV	___ ___ ___ ___ ___	/ /	___ ___ ___ ___
Psychosocial	I, II, III, IV	___ ___ ___ ___ ___	/ /	___ ___ ___ ___
ACT Team	I, II, III, IV	___ ___ ___ ___ ___	/ /	___ ___ ___ ___
Medication Only	I, II, III, IV	___ ___ ___ ___ ___	/ /	___ ___ ___ ___
Opiate Replacement	I, II, III, IV	___ ___ ___ ___ ___	/ /	___ ___ ___ ___
Residential/Inpatient				
Crisis Intervention	I, II, III, IV	___ ___ ___ ___ ___	/ /	___ ___ ___ ___
Crisis Stabilization	I, II, III, IV	___ ___ ___ ___ ___	/ /	___ ___ ___ ___
Hospitalization	I, II, III, IV	___ ___ ___ ___ ___	/ /	___ ___ ___ ___
Medical Detox	I, II, III, IV	___ ___ ___ ___ ___	/ /	___ ___ ___ ___
Nonmedical Detox	I, II, III, IV	___ ___ ___ ___ ___	/ /	___ ___ ___ ___
Residential (–90 days)	I, II, III, IV	___ ___ ___ ___ ___	/ /	___ ___ ___ ___
Residential (90+ days)	I, II, III, IV	___ ___ ___ ___ ___	/ /	___ ___ ___ ___
Supportive Housing	I, II, III, IV	___ ___ ___ ___ ___	/ /	___ ___ ___ ___
Other _____	I, II, III, IV	___ ___ ___ ___ ___	/ /	___ ___ ___ ___
Other _____	I, II, III, IV	___ ___ ___ ___ ___	/ /	___ ___ ___ ___

ADDITIONAL INFORMATION ON _____ (Program's Name)

Observed Qualities

Accessibility of Services	Yes No	Comments:
Integrated Treatment	Yes No	Comments:
Competency Based View	Yes No	Comments:
Treatment Flexibility	Yes No	Comments:
Variable Stays	Yes No	Comments:

Willingness to Add/Expand Co-Occurring Tx Services: Yes No

What Types of Services: _____

What Is Needed to Add/Expand the Services: _____

Additional Comments:
_____
_____

[a]C/O/D – co-occurring disorder

[b]Ind – Individual; Gp = Group; CM = _____; Fam = Family; Med = Medical

[c]FTE = full-time equivalents

[d]H = housing; F = financial; M = medical; E = employment

EXISTING COMMUNITY CO-OCCURRING DISORDERS TREATMENT RESOURCES

Existing Continuum of Care

Components	Currently	Subgroups	Services[a] Ind Gp CM Fam Med	Total #FTEs/Static/Annual[b]	Community Links[c] H F M E
Pretreatment					
Prevention	Yes No	I, II, III, IV	— — — — —	/ /	| | | |
Outreach	Yes No	I, II, III, IV	— — — — —	/ /	| | | |
Early Intervention	Yes No	I, II, III, IV	— — — — —	/ /	| | | |
Outpatient					
Intensive Day	Yes No	I, II, III, IV	— — — — —	/ /	| | | |
Intensive Tx	Yes No	I, II, III, IV	— — — — —	/ /	| | | |
Outpatient Tx	Yes No	I, II, III, IV	— — — — —	/ /	| | | |
Psychosocial	Yes No	I, II, III, IV	— — — — —	/ /	| | | |
ACT Team	Yes No	I, II, III, IV	— — — — —	/ /	| | | |
Medication Only	Yes No	I, II, III, IV	— — — — —	/ /	| | | |
Opiate Replacement	Yes No	I, II, III, IV	— — — — —	/ /	| | | |
Residential/Inpatient					
Crisis Intervention	Yes No	I, II, III, IV	— — — — —	/ /	| | | |
Crisis Stabilization	Yes No	I, II, III, IV	— — — — —	/ /	| | | |
Hospitalization	Yes No	I, II, III, IV	— — — — —	/ /	| | | |
Medical Detox	Yes No	I, II, III, IV	— — — — —	/ /	| | | |
Nonmedical Detox	Yes No	I, II, III, IV	— — — — —	/ /	| | | |
Residential (–90 days)	Yes No	I, II, III, IV	— — — — —	/ /	| | | |
Residential (90+ days)	Yes No	I, II, III, IV	— — — — —	/ /	| | | |
Supportive Housing	Yes No	I, II, III, IV	— — — — —	/ /	| | | |
Other ___		I, II, III, IV	— — — — —	/ /	| | | |
Other ___		I, II, III, IV	— — — — —	/ /	| | | |

Assessment of Current Quality of Services and Expansion Possibilities

Observed Qualities of Current Co-Occurring Treatment Services

Accessibility
of Services   Comments:

Integrated
Treatment   Comments:

Competency
Based View   Comments:

Treatment
Flexibility   Comments:

Variable
Stays   Comments:

Willingness to Add/Expand Co-Occurring Tx Services: Yes   No

What Types of Services: _____

What Is Needed to Add/Expand the Services: _____

_____

Additional Comments:

_____

_____

[a]C/O/D – co-occurring disorder

[b]Ind – Individual; Gp = Group; CM = _____ ; Fam = Family; Med = Medical

[c]FTE = full-time equivalents

[d]H = housing; F = financial; M = medical; E = employment

Appendix B

Interview Questions and Sample Applicant Evaluation Form

The purpose of this appendix is to provide the reader with sample inter-view questions and several case examples that can be used when interview-ing candidates for clinical positions that provide treatment services to indi-viduals with co-occurring disorders. The clinical questions are designed to require applicants to demonstrate that they have the knowledge, interest, and philosophical base needed to provide effective treatment services for individuals with co-occurring disorders. Case examples are designed to al-low applicants to demonstrate their ability to make pertinent observations and assessments of individuals with substance use and psychiatric symp-toms and develop initial treatment plans. A case example is included for each of the four subgroups of this population. A set of questions are also presented with the case examples. These interview questions and case ex-amples can be used as presented or modified to meet the specific needs of a treatment program. Chapter 6 presents detailed information about conduct-ing interviews of applicants for co-occurring disorders treatment positions.

EXAMPLE INTERVIEW QUESTIONS

1. Why are you interested in a clinical position that provides treatment services to individuals with co-occurring disorders?
2. What theoretical or philosophical base do you think is most effec-tive for working with individuals with co-occurring disorders and how is your theoretical or philosophical base similar or different from that base?
3. What assets do you think a clinician needs to be effective with indi-viduals with co-occurring disorders? Which of these do you think are the most important? Which of these would be the easiest for you to perform and which would be the most difficult?

4. What type of substance use and mental disorders would you expect to encounter when working with individuals with co-occurring disorders?

5. Many substance-using individuals experience mental health symptoms as a result of this use. What methods have you found useful in helping to differentiate substance-induced disorders from true co-occurring disorders?

6. How would you define integrated treatment and what would be your thoughts on its benefits for individuals with co-occurring disorders?

7. How would you modify traditional substance abuse treatment for individuals who have both a serious mental disorder and a substance use disorder?

8. How would you modify traditional mental health treatment for individuals who also had a substance use disorder?

9. Many clients with whom you may work will exhibit Axis II personality disorders or traits. In your experience, what impact do these disorders or traits have on treatment and what methods have you found effective in dealing with them?

10. What type of clinical supervision do you think you would need to be most effective working with individuals with co-occurring disorders?

CASE EXAMPLES

Subgroup I (Low Substance Use/Low Psychiatric Symptoms)

Mary is a twenty-year-old female who has come to your program because of insistence that she do so by her parents, with whom she lives. The client was arrested for possession of marijuana after a car in which she was a passenger was pulled over by the police for failing to yield; the officer smelled marijuana and searched the car. The client acknowledges that she and her friend were smoking marijuana and that they shouldn't have been in a car in their condition. Mary also acknowledges that she smokes marijuana a couple of times per month and also drinks alcohol several times a month. She states that marijuana makes her feel calmer. She has never lived away from home and attends the local community college. Mary also reports always having difficulty in school because she has trouble taking tests. Her intelligence level appears normal and she seems fairly honest in her responses.

Subgroup II (Low Substance Use/High Psychiatric Symptoms)

William is a thirty-year-old male who has been referred to your program by his pretrial probation officer for an assessment. He had been arrested for assault and possession of marijuana. The incident occurred when the client, who had been panhandling, got into a verbal dispute with a passerby. The verbal dispute increased in intensity and the client physically assaulted the other individual. Other individuals passing by quickly interceded and no one was seriously injured. The police were called and William was arrested. During the arrest process a small amount of marijuana was found on the client's person. William has a history of minor criminal charges that includes drinking in public, trespassing, and a previous marijuana possession conviction. William is unclear in his responses and is very suspicious of your assessment questions. The client's level of intelligence is also unclear. He is unkempt and has poor personal hygiene.

Subgroup III (High Substance Use/Low Psychiatric Symptoms)

Martha is a twenty-six-year-old female who is referred to your program because of her second driving while intoxicated (DWI) charge. The client's first DWI charge occurred three years ago. Her blood alcohol concentration (BAC) at the time of the first DWI was .18 and her most recent BAC was .22. Martha attended college for about a year after high school and has worked marginal jobs since dropping out. On one occasion she lost her apartment and lived in her car for about a month before she found another apartment. The client's family lives in the area but she has little contact with them. Martha reports that she comes from a very dysfunctional family. She doesn't appear to have any close friends and she stated she hasn't had a date in nearly a year. The client reports that she normally goes home after work, watches TV, and has a beer. Martha appears to be of average or above-average intelligence, and in general is pleasant and presents in a non-demanding manner. Her presentation, however, is slow in thought, movement, and speech.

Subgroup IV (High Substance Use/High Psychiatric Symptoms)

George is a thirty-one-year-old male who has been referred to your program by an outreach worker for the homeless. The client has a long history of significant periods of homelessness. He is currently staying nights in an abandoned house and panhandles during the day. George was discharged two months ago from a psychiatric unit to the local shelter, but left after two days because he didn't feel safe there. The client is an only child and his parents are both deceased. He is not really interested in treatment services, but the local police and merchants, who have known him over the years, asked the homeless persons case manager to try to get him some help because they are concerned for his welfare. George smells of marijuana and alcohol and seems very odd and suspicious of you. It appears that he has not changed his clothes or taken a bath in a very long time. He seems distracted when you are talking to him and some of his answers to your questions don't make sense. George asks you to give him some money to pay for something to eat.

ASSESSMENT AND TREATMENT PLANNING QUESTIONS

The following questions can be used to demonstrate an applicant's level of skill in making assessment and treatment planning decisions when using the previous or other case examples.

1. What additional information would you like to have about the client and why?
2. Where or from whom might you obtain this information?
3. What is the likelihood you will get this information?
4. Discuss your initial Axis I and Axis II diagnostic impressions.
5. To which subgroup does this client belong?
6. Discuss your treatment goals based on these initial diagnostic impressions.
7. What services will ultimately be needed to achieve these goals and what parts of the continuum of care will have to be used?
8. How long do you think it will take to achieve these goals?
9. What client strengths can be used to achieve these goals?
10. Where would you start? What type of treatment do you think you can get the client to participate in at this time?

APPLICANT ASSESSMENT FORM

This form allows interviewers to make comparisons of different applicants based on seven criteria, which were explored in the interview questions and case examples found in this appendix. Each applicant can be rated as high, medium, or low in each area. This form can be used by each interviewer or used as a consensus form of the interview team. Program administrators could choose to place more importance on certain criteria depending on their clinical needs.

Applicant	Experience Level	Interest Level	Knowledge Level	Assessment Skills	Tx Planning Skills	Tx Skills (Axis I)	Tx Skills (Axis II)	General Comments
	H M L	H M L	H M L	H M L	H M L	H M L	H M L	
	H M L	H M L	H M L	H M L	H M L	H M L	H M L	
	H M L	H M L	H M L	H M L	H M L	H M L	H M L	
	H M L	H M L	H M L	H M L	H M L	H M L	H M L	
	H M L	H M L	H M L	H M L	H M L	H M L	H M L	
	H M L	H M L	H M L	H M L	H M L	H M L	H M L	

Appendix C

Training Needs Assessment Form

The purpose of this appendix is to provide the reader with a self-reported needs assessment of co-occurring disorders clinical skills that can be used to identify training needs and training interests. The needs assessment can be completed by each individual staff member or can be used as a composite view of staff by supervisory or management personnel. It covers all essential knowledge and skills areas needed by clinical staff working with this population (see Chapter 6). The needs assessment form asks each individual to rate his or her current level of knowledge and skills in each training area by using a five-point scale that ranges from low to high. The form asks each individual to use this same scale to rate his or her level of interest in receiving training on each topic. Measuring interest levels helps determine the level of motivation activities needed in any planned training activities. Chapter 7 discusses how this needs assessment can be used to develop staff training programs.

CO-OCCURRING DISORDERS CLINICAL NEEDS SURVEY

Please rate each of the following topics according to:

1. Your current skill and knowledge level of a topic
2. Your level of interest in receiving training in that topic

Topic	Low		Moderate		High
History of Dual-Diagnosis Treatment					
Knowledge and Skill Level	1	2	3	4	5
Training Interest	1	2	3	4	5
Nature, Prevalence, and Subgroups					
Knowledge and Skill Level	1	2	3	4	5
Training Interest	1	2	3	4	5
Assessment Techniques and Treatment Planning					
Knowledge and Skill Level	1	2	3	4	5
Training Interest	1	2	3	4	5
Individual and Case Management Interventions					
Knowledge and Skill Level	1	2	3	4	5
Training Interest	1	2	3	4	5
Group Interventions					
Knowledge and Skill Level	1	2	3	4	5
Training Interest	1	2	3	4	5
Family Interventions					
Knowledge and Skill Level	1	2	3	4	5
Training Interest	1	2	3	4	5
Treatment Outcome Measures and Standards					
Knowledge and Skill Level	1	2	3	4	5
Training Interest	1	2	3	4	5

THANK YOU

References

American Psychiatric Association (1980). *Diagnostic and Statistical Manual of Mental Disorders,* Third Edition. Washington, DC: Author.

American Society of Addiction Medicine (2001). *Patient Placement Criteria for the Treatment of Substance-Related Disorders,* Second Edition, Revised. Chevy Chase, MD: Author.

Ball, J.C. and Ross, A. (Eds.) (1991). *The Effectiveness of Methadone Maintenance Treatment: Patients, Programs, Services and Outcome.* New York: Springer-Verlag.

Bartels, S.J. and Drake, R.E. (1996). Residential treatment for dual diagnosis. *Journal of Nervous and Mental Disease,* 184, 379-381.

Bartels, S.J. and Thomas, W.N. (1991). Lessons from a pilot residential treatment program for people with dual diagnoses of severe mental illness and substance use disorder. *Psychosocial Rehabilitation Journal,* 15(2), 19-30.

Bennett, M.E., Bellack, A.S., and Gearson, J.S. (2000). Treating substance abuse in schizophrenia: An initial report. *Journal of Substance Abuse Treatment,* 20, 163-175.

Bernard, J.M. and Goodyear, R.K. (1992). *Fundamentals of Clinical Supervision.* Boston, MA: Allyn & Bacon.

Biederman, J. (1999). Pharmacotherapy of attention-deficit/hyperactivity disorder reduces risk for substance use disorder. *Pediatrics,* 104(2), 20.

Blackwell, J., Beresford, J., Lambert, S. (1988). Patterns of alcohol use and psychiatric inpatient admissions. *Journal of Substance Abuse Treatment,* 5, 27-31.

Blumenthal, S.J. (1988). A guide to risk factors, assessment, and treatment of suicidal patients. *Medical Clinics of North America,* 72(4), 937-971.

Bond, G.R., McDonel, E.C., Miller, L.D., and Pensec, M. (1991). Assertive community treatment and reference groups: An evaluation of their effectiveness for young adults with serious mental illness and substance abuse problems. *Psychosocial Rehabilitation Journal,* 15(2), 31-43.

Borders, L. and Leddick, G. (1987). *Handbook of Clinical Supervision.* Alexandria, VA: American Association of Counseling and Development.

Burnam, M.A., Morton, S.C., McGlynn, E.A., Petersen, L.P., Stecher, B.M., Hayes, C., and Vaccaro, J.V. (1995). An experimental evaluation of residential and non-residential treatment for dually diagnosed homeless adults. *Journal of Addictive Disease,* 14(4), 111-134.

Case, N. (1991). The dual-diagnosis patient in a psychiatric day treatment program: A treatment failure. *Journal of Substance Abuse Treatment,* 8, 69-73.

Caton, C.L.M., Gralnick, A., Bender, S., and Simon, R. (1989). Young chronic patients and substance abuse. *Hospital and Community Psychiatry,* 40(10), 1037-1040.

Center for Mental Health Services (1998). Managed Care Initiative Panel on Co-Occurring Disorders: Co-Occurring Psychiatric and Substance Disorders in Managed Care Systems: Standards or Care, Practice Guidelines, Workforce Competencies, and Training Curricula. Rockville, MD: SAMHSA.

Center for Substance Abuse Treatment (1994a). *Assessment and Treatment of Patients with Coexisting Mental Illness and Alcohol and Other Drug Abuse: Treatment Improvement Protocol (TIP) Series #9.* Washington, DC: DHHS Publication No. (SMA) 94-2078.

Center for Substance Abuse Treatment (1994b). *Confidentiality of Patient Records for Alcohol and Other Drug Treatment. Treatment Assistance Publication (TAP) Series #13.* Washington, DC: DHHS Publication No. (SMA) 95-3018.

Center for Substance Abuse Treatment (1999). *Welfare Reform and Substance Abuse Treatment Confidentiality: General Guidance for Reconciling Need to Know and Privacy. Treatment Assistance Publication (TAP) Series #24.* Washington, DC: DHHS Publication No. (SMA) 99-3332.

Center for Substance Abuse Treatment (2005). *Substance Abuse Treatment for Persons with Co-Occurring Disorders: Treatment Improvement Protocol (TIP) Series #42.* Washington, DC: DHHS Publication No. (SMA) 05-3992.

Cloninger, C.R. (1987). Neurogenic adaptive mechanisms in alcoholism. *Science,* 236, 410-416.

Drake, R.E., McHugo, G.J., Clark, R.E., Teague, G.B., Xie, H., Miles, K., Ackerson, T.H. (1998). Assertive community treatment for patients with co-occurring severe mental illness and substance use disorder. *American Journal of Orthopsychiatry,* 68(2), 201-215.

Drake, R.E., McHugo, G.J., and Noordsy, D.L. (1993). Treatment of alcoholism among schizophrenic outpatients: 4-year outcomes. *American Journal of Psychiatry,* 150(2), 328-329.

Drake, R.E., Osher, F., and Wallach, M. (1991). Homelessness and dual diagnosis. *American Psychologist,* 46, 1149-1158.

Drake, R.E. and Wallach, M.A. (1989). Substance abuse among the chronic mentally ill. *Hospital and Community Psychiatry,* 40(10), 1041-1045.

Drug and Alcohol Serivces Information System (2002). *National Admissions to Substance Abuse Treatment Services.* DASIS Series: S-17, DHHS Publication No. (SMA) 02-3727. Rockville, MD: SAMHSA.

Durell, J., Lechtenberg, B., Corse, S., and Frances, R.J. (1993). Intensive case management of persons with chronic mental illness who abuse substances. *Hospital and Community Psychiatry,* 44, 415-416.

Fischer, P.J. (1991). *Alcohol, Drug Abuse, and Mental Health Problems Among Homeless Persons: A Review of the Literature.* Rockville, MD: National Institute of Mental Health.

Gerstein, D.R., Johnson, R.A., Harwood, H.J., Suter, N., and Malloy, K. (1994). Evaluating Recovery Services: The California Drug and Alcohol Treatment Assessment (CALDATA). Sacramento: California Department of Alcohol and Drug Programs.

Gossop, M., Marsden, J., Stewart, D., Edwards, C., Lehmann, P., Wilson, A., and Segar, G. (1997). The national treatment outcome research study in the United Kingdom: Six-month follow-up outcomes. *Psychology of Addictive Behaviors,* 11(4), 324-337.

Hanson, M., Kramer, T.H., and Gross, W. (1990). Outpatient treatment of adults with coexisting substance use and mental disorders. *Journal of Substance Abuse Treatment,* 7, 109-116.

Hartel, D.M., Schoenbaum, E.E., Selwyn, P.A., Kline, J., Davenny, K., Klein, R.S., and Friedland, G.H. (1995). Heroin use during methadone maintenance treatment: The importance of methadone dose and cocaine use. *American Journal of Public Health,* 85, 83-88.

Hellerstein, D.J., Rosenthal, R.N., and Miner, C.R. (1995). A prospective study of integrated outpatient treatment for substance-abusing schizophrenic patients. *American Journal on Addictions,* 4, 33-42.

Hendrickson, E.L. (1988). Treating the dually diagnosed (mental disorder/substance abuse) client. *TIE Lines,* 5, 1-4.

Hendrickson, E. and Schmal, M. (1993). Dual Disorder Page. *TIE Lines,* 10(3), 11.

Hendrickson, E. and Schmal, M. (2000). Dual Diagnosis Treatment: An 18-Year Perspective. Paper presented at MISA Conference sponsored by MCP-Hahnemann University, Philadelphia, PA.

Hendrickson, E.L., Schmal, M.S., and Ekleberry, S. (2004). *Treating Co-Occurring Disorders: A Handbook for Mental Health and Substance Abuse Professionals.* Binghamton, NY: The Haworth Press.

Hendrickson, E.L., Schmal, M.S., Ekleberry, S., and Bullock, J. (1999). Supervising staff treating the dually diagnosed. *The Counselor,* March/April, 18-22.

Hendrickson, E. L., Stith, S.M., and Schmal, M.S. (1995). Predicting treatment outcome for seriously mentally ill substance abusers in an outpatient dual diagnosis group. *Continuum: Developments in Ambulatory Mental Health Care,* 2(4), 271-289.

Herman, M., Galanter, M., and Lifshultz, H. (1991). Combined substance abuse and psychiatric disorders in homeless and domiciled patients. *American Journal of Drug and Alcohol Abuse,* 17, 415-422.

Hien, D., Zimberg, S., Weisman, S., First, M., and Ackerman, S. (1997). Dual diagnosis subtypes in urban substance abuse and mental health clinics. *Psychiatric Services,* 48(8), 1058-1063.

Hoffman, N.G., Harrison, P.A., and Belille, C.A. (1983). Alcoholics anonymous after treatment: Attendance and abstinence. *International Journal of Addictions,* 18, 311-318.

Hoffman, N.G. and Miller, N.S. (1992). Treatment outcomes for abstinence-based programs. *Psychiatric Annals,* 22(8), 402-408.

Hubbard, R.L., Craddock, S.G., Flynn, P.M., Anderson, J., and Etherridge, R.M. (1997). Overview of 1-year follow-up outcomes in the drug abuse treatment outcome study (DATOS). *Psychology of Addictive Behaviors,* 11(4), 261-278.

Hubbard, R.L., Marsden, M.E., Rachal, J.V., Harwood, H.J., Cavanaugh, E.R., and Ginsburg, H.M. (1989). Drug Abuse Treatment: A National Study of Effectiveness. Chapel Hill, NC: University of North Carolina Press.

Inspector General, Health and Human Services (1995). Services to Persons with Co-Occurring Mental Health and Substance Abuse Disorders: Provider Perspectives. Washington, DC: Health and Human Services.

Jacobi, K.S., Hendrickson, E.L., and Wallace, C. (2002). Lessons learned: Implementing substance abuse treatment services for welfare reform recipients. *The Counselor,* February (3), 20-27.

Kessler, R.C., Nelson, C.B., McGonagle, K.A., Edlund, M.J., Frank, R.G., and Leaf, P.J. (1994). The epidemiology of co-occurring addictive and mental disorders: Implications for prevention and service utilization. *American Journal of Orthopsychiatry,* 66(1), 17-31.

Kofoed, L., Kania, J., Walsh, T., and Atkinson, R.M. (1986). Outpatient treatment of patients with substance abuse and coexisting psychiatric disorders. *American Journal of Psychiatry,* 143, 867-872.

Lee, G. (1982). Social work training versus alcoholism counselor training. *Oregon NASW Newsletter,* October, 1-2.

Lehman, A.F. (1996). Heterogeneity of person and place: Assessing co-occurring addictive and mental disorders. *American Journal of Orthopsychiatry,* 66, 32-41.

Levin, E.R., Evans, S.M., McDowell, D.M., and Kleber, H.D. (1998). Methylphenidate treatment for cocaine abusers with adult attention-deficit/hyperactivity disorder: A pilot study. *Journal of Clinical Psychiatry,* 59(6), 300-305.

Machell, D.F. (1987). Obligations of a clinical supervisor. *Alcoholism Treatment Quarterly,* 8(1), 69-86.

Maisto, S.A., Carey, K.B., Carey, M.P., Purnine, D.M., and Barnes, K.L. (1999). Methods of changing patterns of substance use among individuals with co-occurring schizophrenia and substance use disorder. *Journal of Substance Abuse Treatment,* 17(3), 221-227.

Mammo, A. and Weinbaum, D.F. (1993). Some factors that influence dropping out from outpatient alcoholism treatment facilities. *Journal of Studies of Alcohol,* 45, 359-362.

McCollum, E.E. and Trepper, T.S. (2001). *Family Solutions for Substance Abuse: Clinical and Counseling Approaches.* Binghamton, NY: The Haworth Press.

McCrady, B.S., Noel, N.E., Abrams, D.B., Stout, R.L., Nelson, H.F., and Hay, W.M. (1986). Comparative effectiveness of three types of spouse involvement in out-patient behavioral alcoholism treatment. *Journal of Studies on Alcohol,* 47, 459-467.

McDaniel, S., Weber, T., and McKeever, J. (1983). Multiple theoretical approaches to supervision: Choices in family therapy training. *Family Process,* 22, 491-500.

Mee-Lee, D. (1994). Managed care and dual diagnosis. In Miller, N.S. (Ed.), *Treating Coexisting Psychiatric and Addictive Disorders* (pp. 257-269). Center City, MN: Hazelden Educational Materials.

Meisler, N., Blankertz, L., Santos, A.B., and McKay, C. (1997). Impact of assertive community treatment on homeless persons with co-occurring severe psychiatric and substance use disorders. *Community Mental Health Journal,* 33(2), 113-122.

Metropolitan Washington Council of Governments (1995). *The Treatment of Dual Diagnosis: A Policy Report for the Washington Metropolitan Region.* Washington, DC.

Mierlak, D., Galanter, M., Spivack, N., Dermatis, H., Jurewica, E., and De Leon, G. (1998). Modified therapeutic community treatment for homeless dually diagnosed men. *Journal of Substance Abuse Treatment,* 15(2), 117-121.

Minkoff, K. (1989). An integrated treatment model for dual diagnosis of psychosis and addiction. *Hospital and Community Psychiatry,* 40, 1031-1036.

Minkoff, K. (1993). Intervention strategies for people with dual diagnosis. *Innovations and Research,* 2(4), 11-17.

Minkoff, K. and Cline, C.A. (2004). Changing the world: The design and implementation of comprehensive continuous integrated systems of care for individuals with co-occurring disorders. *Psychiatric Clinics of North America,* 27(4), 727-743.

Mueser, K.T., Drake, R.E., Clark, R.E., Mchugo, G.J., Mercer-McFadden, C., and Ackerson, T.H. (1995). *Toolkit for Evaluating Substance Abuse in Persons with Severe Mental Illness.* Concord, NH: New Hampshire-Dartmouth Psychiatric Research Center.

Nace, E.P. (1989). Substance use disorders and personality disorders: Comorbidity. *The Psychiatric Hospital,* 20(2), 65-69.

National Association of State Alcohol and Drug Abuse Directors (2002). Alcohol and Other Drug Treatment Effectiveness: A Review of State Outcome Studies. Washington, DC: Author.

O'Farrel, T.J. (1989). Marital and family therapy in alcoholism treatment. *Journal of Substance Abuse Treatment,* 6, 23-29.

Onken, L.S., Blaine, J., Genser, S., and Horton, A.M. (Eds.) (1997). *Treatment of Drug-Dependent Individuals with Comorbid Mental Disorders.* NIDA Research Monograph 172, NIH Publication No. 97-4172. Rockville, MD: National Institute on Drug Abuse.

Ornstein, P. and Cherepon, J.A. (1985). Demographic variables as predictors of alcoholism treatment outcome. *Journal of Studies on Alcohol,* 46, 425-432.

Osher, F.C. and Kofoed, L.L. (1989). Treatment of patients with psychiatric and psychoactive substance abuse disorders. *Hospital and Community Psychiatry,* 40, 1025-1030.

Pepper, B. (1995). A community-client protection system (CCPS) for the 21st century. *TIE Lines,* XIII, 7-9.

Pepper, B., Kirshner, M.C., and Ryglewicz, H. (1981). The young adult chronic patient: Overview of population. *Hospital and Community Psychiatry,* 32, 463-469.

Pepper, B. and Massaro, J. (1992). Trans-Institutionalization: Substance abuse and mental illness in the criminal justice system. *TIE Lines,* 9(2), 1-4.

Pepper, B. and Ryglewicz, H. (1984). The young adult chronic patient: A new focus. In Talbott, J. (Ed.), *The Chronic Mental Patient: Five Years Later* (pp. 154-168). New York: Grune and Stratton.

Powell, B.J., Penick, E.C., Othmer, E., Bingham, S.F., and Rice, A.S. (1982). Prevalence of additional psychiatric syndromes among male alcoholics. *Journal of Clinical Psychiatry,* 43(10), 404-407.

Powell, D.J. and Brodsky, A. (2004). *Clinical Supervision in Alcohol and Drug Abuse Counseling: Principles Models, Methods,* Revised Edition. San Francisco: Jossey-Bass.

Prochaska, J.O., DiClemente, C.C., and Norcross, J.C. (1992). In search of how people change: Applications to addictive behaviors. *American Psychologist,* 47, 1102-1114.

Regier, D.A., Farmer, M.E., Raem, D.S., Locke, B.Z., Keith, S.J., Judd, L.L., and Goodwin, F.K. (1990). Comorbidity of mental disorders with alcohol and other drug abuse. *Journal of American Medical Association,* 246(19), 2511-2518.

Ridgely, M.S., Goldman, H.H., and Talbott, J.A. (1986). *Chronic Mentally Ill Young Adults with Substance Abuse Problems: A Review of Relevant Literature and Creation of a Research Agenda.* Baltimore: University of Maryland School of Medicine.

Ridgely, M.S., Osher, F.C., and Talbott, J.A. (1987). *Chronic Mentally Ill Young Adults with Substance Abuse Problems: Treatment and Training Issues.* Baltimore: University of Maryland School of Medicine.

Ries, R.K. (1993). The dually diagnosed patient with psychotic symptoms. *Journal of Addictive Diseases,* 12(3), 103-122.

Ross, H., Glaser, F., and Germanson, T. (1988). The prevalence of psychiatric disorders in patients with alcohol and other drug problems. *Archives of General Psychiatry,* 45, 1023-1031.

Sandberg, C., Greenberg, W.M., and Birkmann, J.C. (1991). Drug-free treatment selection for chemical abusers: A diagnostic-based model. *American Journal of Orthopsychiatry,* 61(3), 358-371.

Schuckit, M.A. (1985). The clinical implications of primary diagnostic groups among alcoholics. *Archives of General Psychiatry,* 42, 1043-1049.

Simpson, D.D. and Sells, S.B. (1982). Effectiveness of treatment for drug abuse: An overview of the DARO research program. *Advances in Alcohol and Substance Abuse,* 2, 7-29.

Substance Abuse and Mental Health Services Administration (1994). The National Treatment Improvement Study (NTIES). Rockville, MD: Author.

Substance Abuse and Mental Health Services Administration (1998). Treatment Episode Data (TED): National Admissions to Substance Abuse Treatment Services. Rockville, MD: Author.

Substance Abuse and Mental Health Services Administration (2002). SAMHSA Report to Congress: Report to Congress on the Prevention and Treatment of Co-Occurring Substance Abuse Disorders and Mental Disorders. Rockville, MD: Author.

Tessler, R. and Dennis, D. (1989). A Synthesis of NIMH-Funded Research Concerning Persons Who Are Homeless and Mentally Ill. Rockville, MD: National Institute of Mental Health.

U.S. Public Health Service (2001). Mental Health: A Report of the Surgeon General. Washington, DC: Author.

Vallant, G.E. (1983). *The Natural History of Alcoholism: Causes, Patterns, and Paths to Recovery.* Cambridge, MA: Harvard University Press.

von Bertalanffy, L. (1968). *General Systems Theory.* New York: Braziller.

Weissman, M.M., Myers, J.K., and Harding, P.S. (1980). Prevalence and psychiatric heterogeneity of alcoholism in a United States urban community. *Journal of Studies of Alcohol,* 41(7), 672-681.

Westermeyer, J. (1989). Nontreatment factors affecting treatment outcome in substance abuse. *American Journal of Drug and Alcohol Abuse,* 15(10), 13-29.

Worthington, E.L. (1987). Changes in supervision as counselors and supervisors gain experience: A review. *Professional Psychology,* 18, 189-208.

Index

Order a copy of this book with this form or online at:
http://www.haworthpress.com/store/product.asp?sku=5471

DESIGNING, IMPLEMENTING, AND MANAGING TREATMENT SERVICES FOR INDIVIDUALS WITH CO-OCCURRING MENTAL HEALTH AND SUBSTANCE USE DISORDERS
Blueprints for Action

_____in hardbound at $39.95 (ISBN-13: 978-0-7890-1146-6; ISBN-10: 0-7890-1146-8)

_____in softbound at $24.95 (ISBN-13: 978-0-7890-1147-3; ISBN-10: 0-7890-1147-6)

Or order online and use special offer code HEC25 in the shopping cart.

COST OF BOOKS_____

☐ **BILL ME LATER:** (Bill-me option is good on US/Canada/Mexico orders only; not good to jobbers, wholesalers, or subscription agencies.)

POSTAGE & HANDLING_____
(US: $4.00 for first book & $1.50 for each additional book)
(Outside US: $5.00 for first book & $2.00 for each additional book)

☐ Check here if billing address is different from shipping address and attach purchase order and billing address information.

Signature_____

SUBTOTAL_____

☐ **PAYMENT ENCLOSED: $_____**

IN CANADA: ADD 7% GST_____

☐ **PLEASE CHARGE TO MY CREDIT CARD.**

STATE TAX_____
(NJ, NY, OH, MN, CA, IL, IN, PA, & SD residents, add appropriate local sales tax)

☐ Visa ☐ MasterCard ☐ AmEx ☐ Discover
☐ Diner's Club ☐ Eurocard ☐ JCB

Account # _____

FINAL TOTAL_____
(If paying in Canadian funds, convert using the current exchange rate, UNESCO coupons welcome)

Exp. Date_____

Signature_____

Prices in US dollars and subject to change without notice.

NAME_____

INSTITUTION_____

ADDRESS_____

CITY_____

STATE/ZIP_____

COUNTRY_____ COUNTY (NY residents only)_____

TEL_____ FAX_____

E-MAIL_____

May we use your e-mail address for confirmations and other types of information? ☐ Yes ☐ No We appreciate receiving your e-mail address and fax number. Haworth would like to e-mail or fax special discount offers to you, as a preferred customer. **We will never share, rent, or exchange your e-mail address or fax number.** We regard such actions as an invasion of your privacy.

Order From Your Local Bookstore or Directly From
The Haworth Press, Inc.
10 Alice Street, Binghamton, New York 13904-1580 • USA
TELEPHONE: 1-800-HAWORTH (1-800-429-6784) / Outside US/Canada: (607) 722-5857
FAX: 1-800-895-0582 / Outside US/Canada: (607) 771-0012
E-mail to: orders@haworthpress.com

For orders outside US and Canada, you may wish to order through your local sales representative, distributor, or bookseller.
For information, see http://haworthpress.com/distributors

(Discounts are available for individual orders in US and Canada only, not booksellers/distributors.)

PLEASE PHOTOCOPY THIS FORM FOR YOUR PERSONAL USE.
http://www.HaworthPress.com   BOF04